ROCCO'S
KETO COMFORT FOOD DIET

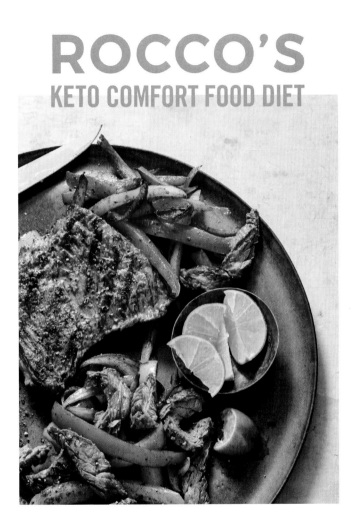

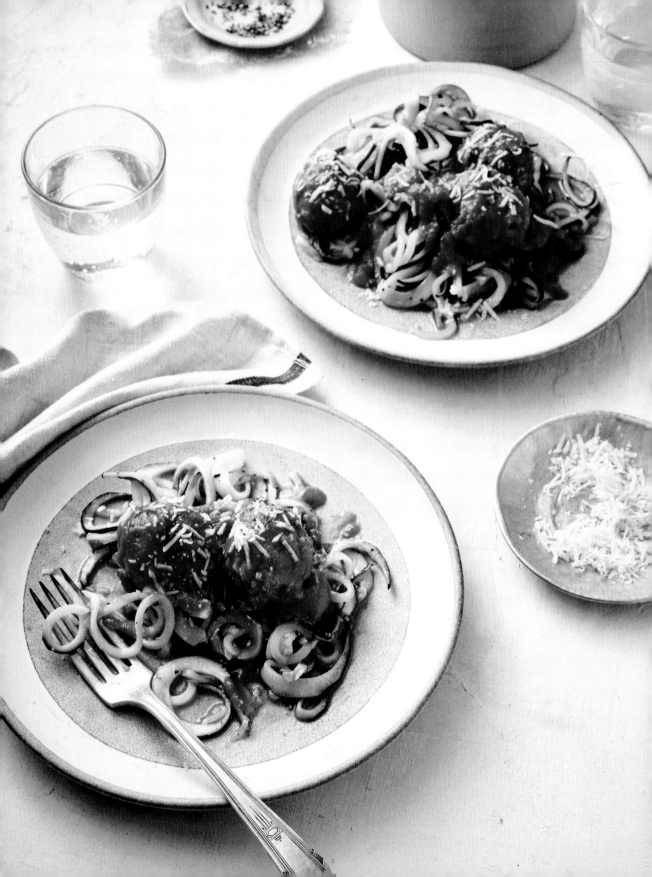

ROCCO'S
KETO COMFORT FOOD DIET

**EAT THE FOODS YOU MISS AND
STILL LOSE UP TO A POUND A DAY**

ROCCO DISPIRITO

RODALE.
NEW YORK

Copyright © 2020 by Rocco DiSpirito
All rights reserved.
Published in the United States by Rodale Books, an imprint of Random House, a division of Penguin Random House LLC, New York.
rodalebooks.com

RODALE and the Plant colophon are registered trademarks of Penguin Random House LLC.

Library of Congress Cataloging-in-Publication Data is available upon request.

ISBN 978-1-9848-2521-6
Ebook ISBN 978-1-9848-2522-3

Printed in the United States of America

Book design by Mia Johnson and Jan Derevjanik
Photographs by Jonathan Pushnik
Cover design by Mia Johnson
Cover photographs by Jonathan Pushnik

10 9 8 7 6 5 4 3 2 1

First Edition

To all my readers over the years who have allowed me into your world to help you live better, healthier, and super fit lives. My work would not be possible without you!

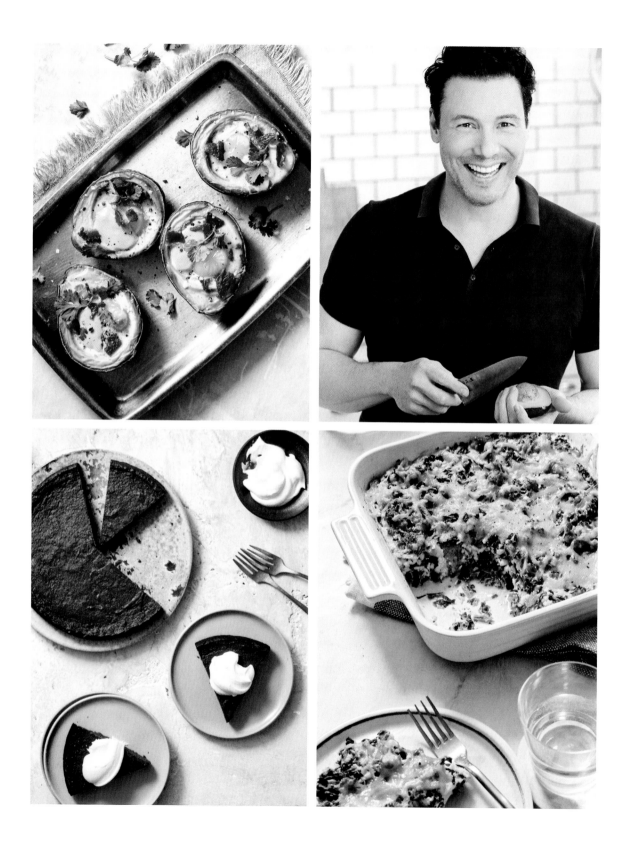

CONTENTS

RECIPE LIST

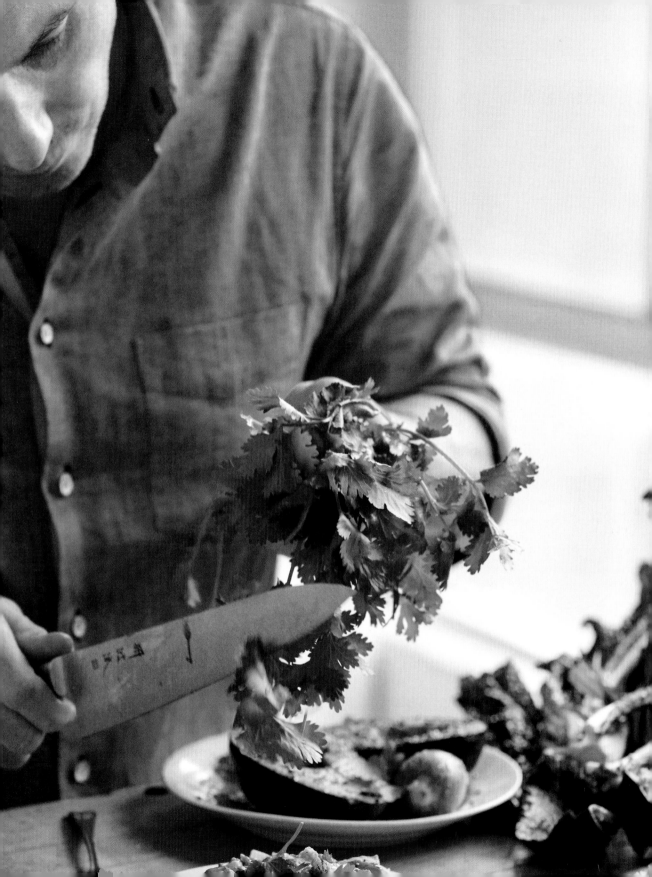

INTRODUCTION

After a long absence of more than a decade, I recently returned to the highly pressurized, intense world of being a head chef at a brand-new New York City restaurant. This can be a grueling process—long days and late nights working to create the perfect menu to satisfy and wow customers.

To get this eatery open and ready for the public, I spent months developing the entire menu. This was a long, painstaking process, but I loved it. I was definitely up for the challenge—it's one of the things I missed most about heading up a restaurant. It was fun creating new dishes and experimenting with flavors. I was using everything I had ever learned—food development, menu creation, and overall kitchen management. I was back in my element. Of course, this process required *a lot* of tasting. Sometimes, though, I wouldn't just taste it, I'd scarf down the whole dish. This is both a perk and a curse. After all, some of the items that ended up on the menu were very rich and not dishes you'd eat daily if you wanted to stay trim and fit.

And so gradually (and inevitably), I began filling out and putting on pounds—to the point that I started wearing baggy shirts and pants. Underneath, I knew I was getting big, and eventually I had to face the music.

One day I woke up, looked at my body in the mirror, and said to myself, "That's it. Enough is enough." I decided to lose that ugly pudge, and I needed to do it fast.

Like everyone else, I had heard about the ketogenic diet. Needing to shed those pounds, I decided to dig deeper, reading and rummaging through all the resources I could find about keto. The ketogenic diet is essentially a fast-results plan for weight loss. You drop pounds quickly—a lot of people have been known to lose up to 10 pounds the first week!—and feel good while on it. You lose inches of fat all over your body. You don't have mood swings caused by spikes in blood sugar, and you rarely feel hungry. And you can eat foods that for many years you've been told not to eat—bacon, eggs, steak, butter, and other fatty foods—because fat, not sugar, is really the ideal fuel for the body.

I remember thinking, what sort of diet magic is this? I can lose weight by eating fat? Cheese? Real cream? Steaks? Bacon? Really? And my most favorite food in the world—butter? What's more, we chefs create and cook with all this stuff backstage in our restaurants all the time. And fat as fuel? I had a lot of that. It was like a dream come true. Count me in!

So I started a keto diet, with hopes of losing shedloads of weight. Initially, I did. But like all my friends, I started getting bored with it. The diet was very limited—no grains, fruits, starchy vegetables, bread, pasta, and legumes like chickpeas and lentils. Eating the same things over and over gave me taste fatigue. I thought I'd eventually crack and wolf down a monster plate of spaghetti. Panic was slowly descending on me.

As a guy who is very good at consuming food, my philosophy is that eating should be enjoyable. Not temporarily enjoyable as in I-had-a-bad-day-so-I'm-going-to-pound-down-a-gallon-of-chocolate-chip-ice-cream. I mean the kind of enjoyable where you love your meals, you get to eat stuff like pizza, you don't feel deprived, and your weight comes off faster than hubcaps stripped from a Lexus parked in a bad neighborhood.

So I wasn't ready to give up.

I started pondering this whole keto-is-boring thing and thinking about how I could turn keto meals into comfort food at its tastiest, especially at a time when my own fat-burning flames needed some fanning. I decided to dust off some strategies that I had used years ago to transform America's favorite comfort foods into deliciously healthy dishes—all with zero bad carbs, zero bad fats, zero sugar, and maximum flavor. These strategies were partly the basis of my bestselling series of *Now Eat This!* books years ago when reducing fat and calories was topical.

Ketogenic diets needed the same big makeover—so that people could eat bread, pancakes, puddings, cookies, cakes with frosting, cheesecake, pizza, tacos, burgers, and more. And none of it could taste like cardboard!

I knew that's what I needed to lose my extra pounds quickly and keep them off—and it's what others needed as well.

The ketogenic diet is medically sound and effective, but any eating plan that feels restrictive cannot work long term. So while there are many books on the keto lifestyle on the market, I knew that no one with the culinary credentials I have or the skill for crafting flavorful dishes had attempted to make over Americans' favorite comfort foods keto-style. I was up for the challenge!

I conjured up about eighty "keto comfort food recipes"—and a diet to go along with them. All the dishes I listed on pages 8 to 9 made the cut. So did the foods I grew up with. As an Italian-American, I love lasagna, spaghetti, and pasta galore. I created keto comfort food versions of these traditional dishes so I could once again enjoy the meals I grew up with. It didn't even feel like keto dieting, and it sure wasn't deprivation.

Along with the recipes, I put all these keto comfort foods into a four-tiered food plan that guarantees you'll stay with a keto diet right down to your target weight—and beyond. Best of all, it includes a maintenance plan called Keto Comfort Phasing that helps you keep that weight off. It's all here. Once you get started, you won't even know you're on a diet, much less a keto diet! And you'll be able to keep your weight off easily.

This book is a completely new, unique, and revolutionary way to use keto dieting to burn fat and keep it off. Here's a look at several of the key weight-control benefits you can expect, all while you enjoy what you are eating.

LOSE WEIGHT SUPER FAST. Ketogenic diets, including my Keto Comfort Food Diet, retrain the body to use fat as an energy source. When you restrict carbs in your diet, your body taps into fat stores and burns them for energy. As a result, it's not unusual to lose up to a pound a day on this diet—as was proven in a test group of dieters who followed my plan.

GET A SLIMMER WAISTLINE. Research into keto diets shows that they trim your waist circumference, otherwise known as belly fat—as well as hip fat—and so will the Keto Comfort Food Diet. Dieters on my plan lost an average of one inch around their waist. Now that's something to look forward to!

SAY GOOD-BYE TO HUNGER PANGS. Studies on keto diets suggest that they reduce ghrelin, a hormone that makes you hungry. What's more, in the fat-burning state called "ketosis," when the body is functioning on a high-fat, moderate-protein, and low-carb diet, your appetite goes down, and cravings are a distant memory. Essentially, you can stay satisfied much longer with my eating plan.

These benefits and others are entirely possible, as long as you stay with it. To do that, you've got to prepare, eat, and enjoy all the delicious keto comfort foods I have for you here. I've taken all the foods you and I love—no matter how bad they might be for us—and turned them into keto comfort food versions that make it easy for you to blast away fat, lose inches, and drop pounds.

As for me, I never had to cheat or fall off the wagon because I was eating these super delicious and super flavorful keto adaptations of my favorite foods. I achieved my weight-loss goal, and my baggy-clothes wardrobe became a casualty.

And I got healthier. My blood pressure, cholesterol, and blood-sugar levels are in the normal ranges now. My mind remained sharp as a whip because the brain loves to run on ketone bodies, by-products of fat breakdown.

My cravings disappeared, too. The higher level of fat in the diet kept me fuller for longer. I never turned "hangry" where I wanted to bite everyone's head off. I'm not tempted by starchy foods, desserts, or sweets, either.

I experienced boundless energy, which is a good thing because now that we've opened the restaurant my schedule is even more grueling than before!

The other good news is that I no longer have to obsess over the endless list of foods I "can't" eat because I can now eat the food that I love. I buy all my food at regular grocery stores and farmers' markets because I get to eat real food. I don't have to purchase processed, packaged diet food that tastes and smells nasty.

I want you to enjoy the wonderful dishes that fit within my real-foods, ketogenic way of eating. With them, you'll drop amazing amounts of weight and inches in no time at all—fast results that will keep you motivated—while enjoying food that won't make you feel deprived. I promise, this brand-new way of doing keto will also improve your health in spectacular ways.

The Keto Comfort Food Diet was definitely something that fit into my lifestyle almost seamlessly. And I know it can work for you, too.

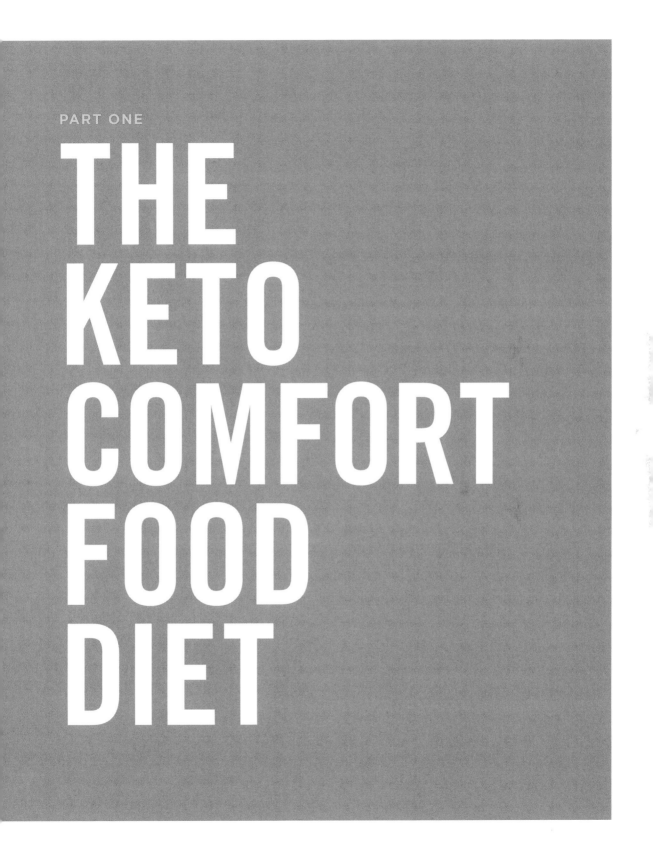

PART ONE

THE KETO COMFORT FOOD DIET

KETO— EVERYTHING YOU NEED TO KNOW

So what is a keto diet?

At its most basic, it's a super-low-carb, high-fat diet. It alters the way your body uses fuel for energy. Rather than burn carbohydrates, your body taps into stored fat for energy, thanks to a process known as ketosis. The result? Rapid weight loss.

Ketosis kicks in because the body is amazing. It knows what it needs and how to get it, and the main thing it wants is fuel. Without fuel, our cells would starve, and well . . . then we're all history.

Normally, most people eat carbs for their daily fuel needs. In fact, carbs are your body's first-line source of energy because they are fast-acting and easily accessible. As long as you eat carbs, your body will convert those carbs into usable energy. Excess carbs, however, are packed away as unsightly fat.

If you deny yourself carbohydrates, the body searches elsewhere for fuel, and the default, or next-line source, is fat. (Protein is the body's least favorite source of energy because protein is required for so many other vital, life-supporting functions in the body.)

As the body switches over to using fat, the liver converts fatty acids into energy-producing molecules called "ketone bodies" and uses them as fuel. This is the state of being in ketosis; it means that your body is burning fat. No longer are you relying on sugar (glucose in the bloodstream) or glycogen (stored carbs in the liver and muscle) for energy; fat is now the source. Your body uses those ketone bodies for energy to power through your day. And not to worry, your body is just as happy using them as it was using glucose or glycogen.

Even your brain likes to run on ketone bodies. They piggyback on a protein called albumin to carry them across the blood-brain barrier—an invisible security system that isolates the brain from the rest of the body, preventing many harmful substances in the blood from breaching and entering the brain. The brain thus readily accepts ketone bodies as an energy source.

When I started on my keto diet, I felt more alert and focused than usual. It was very noticeable. I really wouldn't want to go back. This happens to many keto dieters and is clear evidence that the brain is getting plenty of fuel.

Incidentally, the terms "ketone bodies" and "ketones" are often used interchangeably in discussions around keto diets, but they're slightly different. Ketone bodies, as described above, are alternate forms of fuel the body uses when carbs aren't available; they're a by-product of burning fat. Ketones are chemicals that are always present in the blood. Their levels fluctuate depending on what you eat, how you exercise, and whether you have diseases such as diabetes.

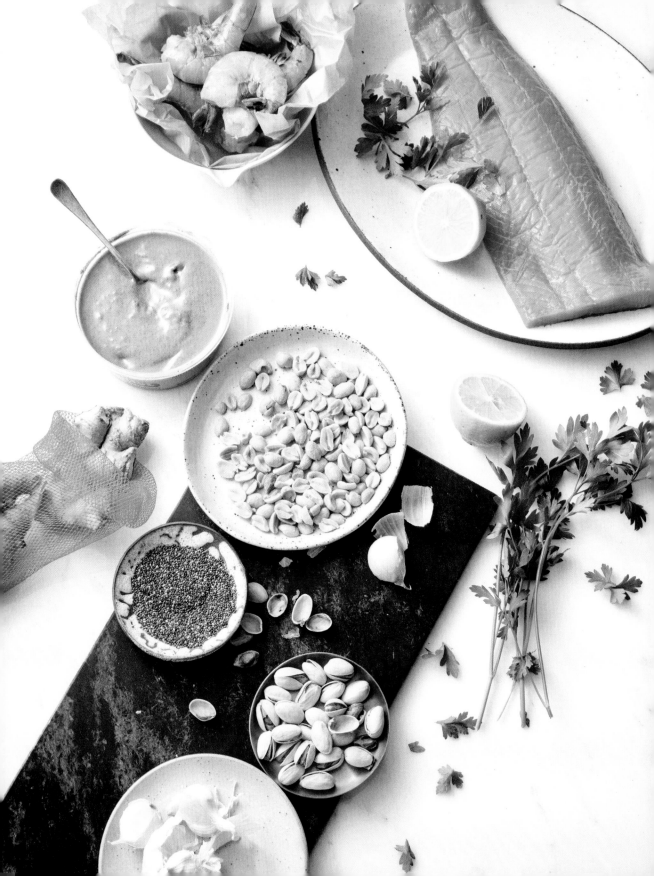

GETTING INTO KETOSIS

After you start a keto diet, your body begins casting off its stored sugar within about 72 hours. At that point, it's forced to draw on fat. After about 4 days to 1 week of restricting carbs and eating more fat, you enter the metabolic state of ketosis, signifying your body has gotten used to burning fat for energy. Everyone is different, but you can expect to lose between ½ pound and 1 pound a day. This is consistent with what I observed in the test group who followed my Keto Comfort Food Diet. Besides rapid fat-burning, ketosis makes you feel less hungry and helps you maintain your lean muscle mass.

To kick your body into ketosis on the Keto Comfort Food Diet, you must do three main things:

1. Severely restrict carbohydrates.

2. Eat moderate amounts of protein.

3. Eat as much saturated fat and monounsaturated fat as it takes to feel satisfied. (Saturated fat is found in meat, dairy foods, and coconut oil; monounsaturated fat is present in nuts, seeds, avocados, and olive oil.)

Thus, a true ketogenic diet like the Keto Comfort Food Diet is low in carbohydrates, moderate in protein, and high in fat. To stay in ketosis, I side with experts on daily nutrient percentages: Roughly 60 to 75 percent of your daily calories should come from fat (60 to 120 grams daily). Five to 10 percent of your calories should come from carbs (20 to 30 grams a day). The remainder, 15 to 30 percent of your daily calories, should be obtained from protein (100 to 150 grams or slightly more, depending on if you work out regularly). These percentages are general guidelines only; they can certainly vary a bit. I won't sentence you to hard time in a bakery if you deviate a little! Simply follow the guidelines provided here and you'll be headed in the right direction.

A FOUR-TIERED PLAN FOR SUCCESS

Looking ahead, you'll see that my plan has four tiers:

TIER 1: THE 3-DAY KETO CLEANSE. This tier kicks off the plan and launches you quickly into ketosis. Men and women who start with this cleanse have dropped between 4 and 8 pounds in 3 days (men will be in the upper range of loss), according to the results in my test group.

TIER 2: THE ACCELERATED 21-DAY KETO COMFORT FOOD DIET. I provide you with 3 weeks of low-calorie and low-carbohydrate meal plans and recipes to continue your rapid and effective weight loss. On this tier, you can burn fat fairly rapidly by clearing sugar and carbs from your body. It incorporates "intermittent fasting" to boost and sustain ketosis.

TIER 3: THE BASIC 21-DAY KETO COMFORT FOOD DIET. You'll up your calories and carbs slightly—plus eat optional keto comfort food desserts—in order to continue your success.

TIER 4: KETO COMFORT PHASING. This is my maintenance plan, which most keto diets neglect to provide. It teaches you how to introduce certain foods back into your diet and helps you stay at your desired weight.

QUICK OVERVIEW OF THE KETO COMFORT FOOD DIET

TIERS	PURPOSE
TIER 1: The Keto Cleanse	A 3-day detox plan to rapidly launch your body into fat-burning. It helps remove sugar and carbohydrates from your system.
TIER 2: The Accelerated Keto Comfort Food Diet	A 21-day plan that is low in calories and carbohydrates. It is designed to sustain rapid fat-burning and employs the strategy of intermittent fasting.
TIER 3: The Basic Keto Comfort Food Diet	A 21-day plan with slightly increased calories and carbohydrates to help you move closer to your goal weight.
TIER 4: Keto Comfort Phasing	A maintenance plan in which you follow ketogenic nutritional principles 4 to 5 days a week, then reintroduce clean carbohydrates and other foods into your lifestyle on the weekends.

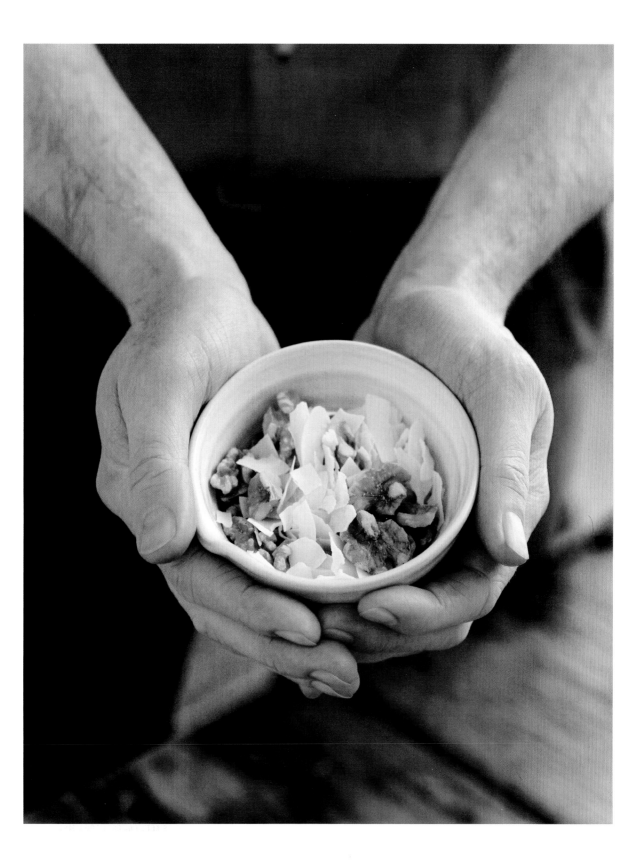

THE KETO LOWDOWN
ON MACRONUTRIENTS

Carbohydrates, protein, and fat are referred to as "macronutrients." That's because they are required in large amounts by the body. Here's a rundown of how they interact on the Keto Comfort Food Diet.

CARBOHYDRATES: WHY YOU DON'T EVEN NEED THEM

As I stated above, ketogenic diets restrict carbohydrates. Is this good or bad? Don't you need them? Don't you risk nutritional deficiencies if you don't eat carbs?

The scientific but surprising answer is no.

I'm going to tell you something hush-hush: Carbohydrates—which include starches and sugar—are not essential. Any nutrient called "essential" means that it is *required* for health and normal body function, and that it has to be obtained from food (because the body can't make it). Essential nutrients include vitamins, minerals, essential fatty acids, and essential amino acids (proteins).

Carbohydrates are not on that list because there is no such thing as an essential carbohydrate. After you eat carbs, they're converted into glucose during digestion, used for energy, or stored as fat. Your body does need some glucose to function, but it doesn't need carbs to get it. If a carb never passed through your lips again, your body would simply convert whatever it can—including protein—into glucose.

If you ate as many starchy carbohydrates as some experts recommend—around 100 grams a day or more—it's virtually impossible to get into ketosis to burn fat or fix a condition such as insulin resistance (meaning your body is unable to use insulin effectively, leading to high blood sugar and, ultimately, diabetes).

Here's something else you should know about eating starchy carbs and too many of them. Research has shown that people who consume a carbohydrate-rich diet are more likely to be diagnosed with depression than those on a diet consisting mostly of protein and vegetables.

This happens because carbohydrates break down into glucose—or sugar—in the body, as I mentioned earlier. Blood sugar can then go up very quickly and drop just as quickly, causing a depressed mood. This link between mood and blood-sugar balance is well known. The more uneven your blood-sugar supply, the more uneven your mood. Who wants to deal with that? Not me!

Happily, though, keto diets are being explored as antidepressant therapy because of their positive effects on the brain. I find this to be fascinating. A 2018 article published in *Neuroscience & Biobehavioral Reviews* stated: "Preclinical studies, case reports and case series have demonstrated antidepressant and mood stabilizing effects of [ketogenic diets]."

Refined carbohydrates such as sugar and white bread are also thought to increase chronic inflammation in the body. That inflammation may affect the brain, leading to depression.

It's true that carbohydrates supply required vitamins and minerals. But there's one category of food that delivers way more of those nutrients than starchy carbs: non-starchy vegetables, which you will eat in copious amounts on the Keto Comfort Food Diet. So end of story: There's no biological reason to eat starchy carbohydrates.

WHAT ABOUT KETO FLU?

During the first week or two of a keto diet, some people experience "keto flu," in which you feel like you're coming down with the actual flu. You're not really getting sick, but you feel the symptoms of flu-like fatigue, head-aches, or brain fog. This might freak you out a little bit as it did me when I experienced it.

The reason this happens on most keto diets is the low dietary level of electrolytes, which are minerals involved in a lot of bodily processes. Common electrolytes are sodium, potassium, calcium, magnesium, and chloride. They regulate hydration, keep your heart beating, and help your muscles contract.

Because my diet is all about "Comfort" with a capital "C," I don't want you to feel uncomfortable about coming down with keto flu. That's why I've populated the Keto Comfort Food Diet with plenty of foods (especially vegetables) that provide electrolytes. For potassium and magnesium, you get to eat lots of leafy greens, cruciferous vegetables like broccoli and cabbage, squash, and the super healthy fat avocado. Calcium is abundant in green leafy vegetables and other low-carb veggies. Water-dense foods like celery, cucumbers, and bell peppers help prevent dehydration and restore electrolytes. When you focus on these foods, they prevent defi-ciencies that contribute to keto flu.

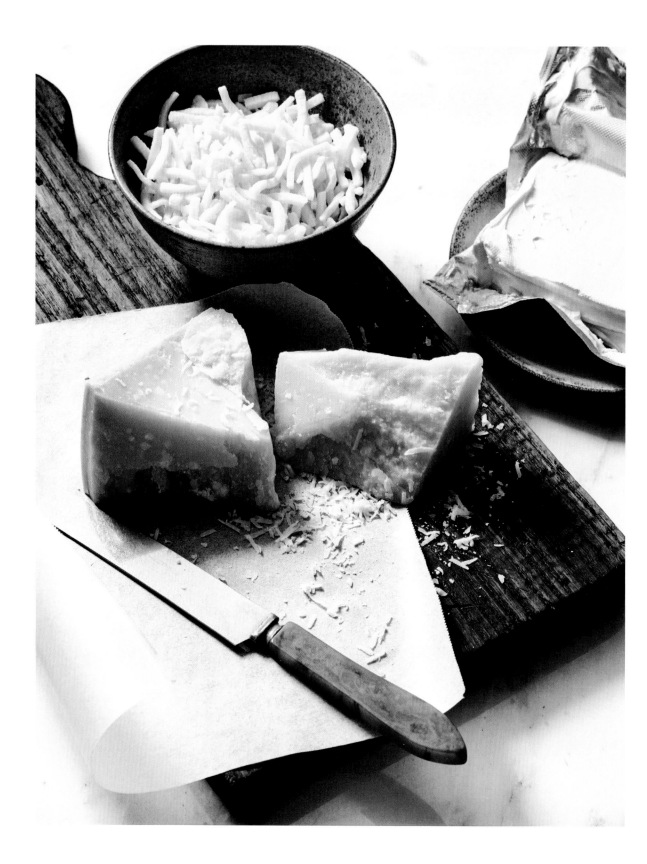

LOW-
CARB
EATING
IS NOT
KETO
DIETING

Keto diets are low-carb, but low-carb diets such as Atkins or South Beach or Paleo are not keto diets. Let me explain why.

1. GRAMS OF CARBOHYDRATES PER DAY. Unless you get your carbs down to 30 to 40 grams a day or under and stay there, then the diet is really not considered "ketogenic"; it's just a simple low-carb diet or even a Paleo diet. On the Atkins diet, for example, you may only be in ketosis during the early phases of the diet, whereas on a keto diet, the goal is to maintain ketosis.

Many diets are simple low-carb plans that allow far more carbs than a keto diet, so your body does not go into ketosis and burn pure fat.

Eating low-carb generally means consuming between 50 and 100 grams of carbs a day. But if you eat upwards of 50 grams of carbs daily, your body will not go into ketosis; in other words, it will not use the breakdown of fat (ketone bodies) for energy. On a low-carb diet, you might still be burning carbs for energy. So basically, you're employing a completely different energy-using pathway when you follow a keto diet.

2. BALANCE OF MACRONUTRIENTS. People who go on a low-carb diet tend to overeat protein (which can turn into glucose and thus prevent ketosis). A keto diet, on the other hand, is a moderate-protein diet. There's simply a lot more emphasis on eating healthy fats and not overdoing it on the protein front (see page 26).

3. FEWER PROCESSED FOODS. Low-carb diets often recommend a lot of processed foods such as low-carb breads, low-carb salad dressings, diet sodas, and bars filled with fake sugars. These foods do not help you achieve nutritional ketosis. Nor are they good for your long-term health. Keto diets, particularly my Keto Comfort Food Diet, emphasize real foods over processed diet foods.

4. THE DAIRY ALLOWANCE. Similar to the keto diet, the Paleo diet eliminates processed foods, legumes, and grains. But one big difference is that you can't eat dairy on Paleo, but you can on the Keto Comfort Food Diet. Personally, I just can't get excited over living a life without cheese. Plus, wasn't the average life span of a Paleolithic caveman between twenty-five and forty?

The bottom line: Using ketone bodies for energy drastically changes your metabolism for more efficient fat-burning. Low-carb diets simply restrict your carb intake. Keto, on the other hand, puts you into nutritional ketosis, the optimal fat-burning state.

THE POWER OF MODERATE PROTEIN

Some people think that on a keto diet you can eat as much protein as you want—that it's a high-protein diet, and that it's okay to pile the whole cow or chicken or pig on your plate. Not true. On a keto diet, it's really important to *not* eat protein by the truckload; you've got to go easy on this macronutrient. If you eat too much protein, beyond what you need, your body converts the excess into glucose (sugar). That works against you—for two reasons.

First, on a keto diet, you want your body to rely solely on fat for fuel, so producing glucose is self-defeating and prevents reliance on fat. Second, if you're insulin-resistant or just looking at a carb makes you gain weight (meaning you're carbohydrate-sensitive), then you certainly don't want to add gas to the fire by overeating protein. For these reasons, the Keto Comfort Food Diet is not a high-protein diet; it is a moderate-protein diet.

Eaten in moderation, protein assists the fat-burning process. At its most basic level, digesting and assimilating protein expends significantly more energy than consuming carbohydrates or fat. The rate at which this energy burn occurs is the "thermic effect of feeding," or TEF. The TEF of carbohydrates is between 5 and 15 percent; this means it takes 5 to 15 calories to burn off 100 calories of foods containing these macronutrients. Fat is between 0 and 5 percent, but it is the number one nutrient for driving ketosis. Protein has the highest TEF—around 20 percent—which is why protein is considered a fat-burning food: one that supports nutritional ketosis.

FAT: NEVER FEAR IT AGAIN

A hallmark of the keto diet is that it is purposely high in fat. Of course, for more than forty years, we've been led to believe that fat is the ultimate food bad guy. The advice went something like this: Eating too much fat will make you fat, clog your arteries, and trigger a heart attack—so eat a lot of low-fat food instead.

Wrong! While we were worried sick over saturated fats and dietary cholesterol and afraid to put oil on our salads or let butter pass through our lips, there was a far more dangerous food baddie lurking around: sugar. Fortunately, world nutrition organizations have come to their senses. They now realize that the amount of sugar we eat—not fat—is responsible for obesity, heart disease, type 2 diabetes, even cancer.

But how did we get so far afield? Since the 1960s, the sugar industry has paid scientists to shed doubt on the link between its product and heart disease, diabetes, and other life-threatening illnesses—a finding unearthed by researchers at the University of California, San Francisco. This cover-up was published in a 2016 issue of the *Journal of the American Medical Association—Internal Medicine.*

It's official: Fat is not the villain. Start wrapping your head around the fact that bacon, butter, and cream aren't our enemies. Those pork rinds? They make a perfectly healthy snack, even a great crust for fish and chicken. Let me add that I do like to emphasize clean, quality fats, too, such as olive oil, coconut oil, avocados, nuts, and seeds.

Furthermore, to stay in ketosis, you've got to consume fat, because that is what your body relies on for fuel. Without fat, it will try its best to burn glycogen (sugar) as its fuel, but that will knock you out of ketosis.

A high-fat diet may help us live longer. A large Canadian study published in 2018 challenged the conventional advice that a low-fat diet is best for heart health and cuts your risk of premature death.

This study from McMaster University involved more than 135,000 people in eighteen countries. It revealed that consuming a higher-fat diet is linked to a reduced risk of early death, whereas consuming a high-carb diet is associated with a greater risk of dying early.

Interesting, right? Not only can you eat fat to lose fat, you can eat it for a long, healthy life.

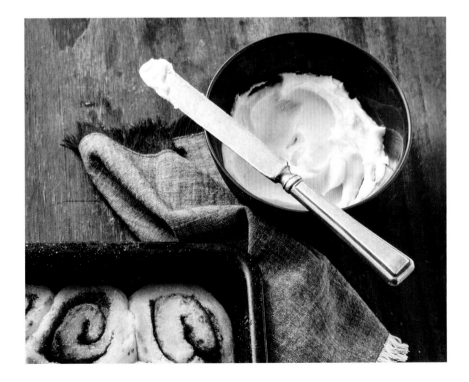

WHAT ELSE DOES SCIENCE SAY?

After you get into ketosis, by sticking to a regimen of mostly fat, protein, and non-starchy vegetables, your body becomes "fat-adapted." This means your muscles are using ketone bodies as fuel and your body has adapted to using stored fat for energy. As long as you keep carbohydrates low enough, this is what the body has to do. The net effect is fat loss.

How well does all this work?

Pretty dramatically, I'd say. Take a look at what science says.

THE KETO DIET TARGETS AND BURNS PURE FAT

Remember that when you curb carbs in your diet, your body starts using up stored carbohydrates (glycogen) for energy. Glycogen is stored with water, so when you restrict carbs, water doesn't have anything to hold on to. This is why carb restriction causes you to lose water weight. Which is fine. Water is weight, too, and after all, who likes bloat?

The keto diet, however, incinerates pure fat. A 2018 Spanish study of 12 obese women found that a keto diet burned off 40 pounds of fat over 4 months—which included nearly 4 pounds of visceral fat. This is a dangerous type of fat that pads our internal organs and is around our waist. Excess visceral fat is associated with serious, sometimes fatal health problems, such as heart disease, type 2 diabetes, and high blood pressure.

THE KETO DIET IS SUPERIOR TO A LOW-CALORIE DIET

A lot of people harp on the value of cutting calories to lose weight, and counting those calories to the point of obsession. (Sure, calorie counting has its place, and it is also important in a keto diet, so I provide calorie counts for the recipes in this book.)

Calorie-counting diets calculate the calories in everything you eat, and they treat all calories the same, whether they come from candy or celery. But clearly not all calories are created equal. We have to consider calorie "quality." The calories from minimally processed foods like vegetables, healthy fats, and proteins—the foods recommended on this diet—are burned off more efficiently than those of poor-quality foods such as candy, sweets, refined sugar, processed foods, and junk foods.

So back to my point: How does traditional calorie counting (quantity) stack up to eating ketogenically (looking at quality and quantity)? Truth be told, not so well.

In one study, researchers compared these two approaches—with a specific focus on belly fat—and discovered that a keto diet induced a greater reduction in body weight (28 pounds overall), waist circumference (5 inches), and pure fat (19 pounds) than the low-calorie diet: 9½ pounds, 1½ inches, and 8 pounds, respectively. Raise your hand: Who likes the idea of losing 28 pounds over losing 9½ pounds? Just about everyone. Again, it's the quality of calories that is important. Quality keto calories help the body burn fat and trim off inches.

THE KETO DIET IS BETTER THAN A LOW-FAT DIET

A low-fat diet is typically structured around slashing dietary fat, with more of your calories coming from protein and carbs. At the time when low-fat-diet guidelines were first promoted (all the way back in 1977), it was assumed that saturated fat was one of the biggest triggers of heart disease, so we were told to follow diets providing less than 10 percent total fat content because this would be so much healthier for our hearts.

This assumption led to the manufacturing of lots of "fat-free" diet products, all unfortunately packed full of refined carbs, sugar, and artificial sweeteners, which are actually associated with heart disease, diabetes, and obesity. So right away, you can see that a low-fat diet laced with sugary processed food wouldn't do your body much good and definitely would not put you in ketosis. A ketogenic diet is thus metabolically far superior to a low-fat diet. Further, when compared with a low-fat diet, the keto diet was a more effective intervention for improving and reversing type 2 diabetes (*Nutrition & Metabolism*, 2008).

THE KETO DIET PRESERVES MUSCLE

Muscle is calorie-burning, fat-burning tissue—the more you have on your body, the more efficient your metabolism. Critics of the keto diet have been quick to point out that maintaining ketosis may strip away precious muscle. But science has not found this to be true. In fact, keto diets consistently attack body fat and leave muscle alone. This was found in a 2018 study of 24 healthy men who followed a keto diet and a weight-training program for 8 weeks. They lost body fat and belly fat while maintaining muscle. This study hinted at the idea that weight training while eating ketogenically is a good idea for preserving body-firming muscle. This is all great news if you're a regular exerciser (we all should be in that club!).

You've heard it, I've heard it: The hard part about weight loss is keeping it off. Well, the truth is, it really isn't all that hard if you adhere to keto dieting. A 2013 British study found that a ketogenic diet produced sustained weight control and improved cardiovascular health when compared with a conventional low-fat diet. To me, these findings are significant and worth applauding. I've always said that weight maintenance, as opposed to weight loss, constitutes the best defense in the war against obesity. A diet can win the battle, but maintenance wins the war—especially when ketogenic nutrition is involved. My Keto Comfort Phasing plan will help you keep your weight off and is something to look forward to.

Bottom line: Science is siding with ketogenic diets as a way to strip the body of fat and control weight.

BEYOND FAT LOSS—AMAZING HEALTH BENEFITS WHEN YOU GO KETO

I started a keto diet in hopes of trimming down fast and getting out of baggy clothes. As I delved into the realm of this approach, I quickly learned that I could do my health—not just my waistline—a world of good. This is why I'd like to see you on the Keto Comfort Food Diet—not just because it will slim you down quickly, not just because the meals are so delicious, but because you deserve to be healthy. My Keto Comfort Food Diet improves heart health, can reverse diabetes, protects the brain, and may even offer a complementary approach to cancer treatment. And with the adjustments I made to make every keto meal enjoyable, it's sustainable. As one of my test subjects told me: "This diet is the first one I've been on where I don't feel like I'm missing my favorite foods. After just several days on it, the diet felt so natural, and I felt amazing."

Here's a brief overview of what I'm talking about.

MAINTAIN A HEALTHY HEART

Many studies and systematic reviews of the keto diet have discovered that it can significantly decrease levels of triglycerides and LDL cholesterol (the bad kind), and raise HDL cholesterol (the good kind). All of these factors help keep the arteries free of plaque buildup, allowing blood to circulate freely to the heart. Keto diets have also been shown to reduce C-reactive protein, a marker of inflammation, which is harmful to the heart and other organs.

A 2010 study published in the *Archives of Internal Medicine* revealed that obese participants who followed a keto diet for 48 weeks not only lost weight but lowered their systolic blood pressure (the top number on the reading) by an average of 5.9 points. Over half the dieters were able to reduce their medication, or stop taking it altogether. The reason for these impressive results is largely due to weight loss, which provides a whole-body benefit and reduces all sorts of metabolic risk factors.

Another reason why keto diets can get your blood pressure under control is that they're high in potassium- and magnesium-loaded foods. Both minerals are involved in regulating blood pressure. A keto diet can even reduce your dependency on blood pressure medications.

DEFEND AGAINST DIABETES

A grim life sentence being dished out to thousands of people every year, diabetes is a disorder of too much sugar (glucose) in the bloodstream. Under normal conditions, glucose feeds the body's cells with the help of the hormone insulin. But in diabetes, either there isn't enough insulin to go around (type 1 diabetes) or the cells have trouble making use of insulin (type 2 diabetes—the most common). The result is that insulin and glucose can't get into cells and thus amass in the blood.

A ketogenic diet is a diabetes fighter. It lowers levels of insulin and blood sugar in the body. When insulin comes down, beneficial fat-burning hormones such as growth hormone kick in, and cortisol, which encourages belly cells to store fat, flatlines.

The keto diet can benefit people with type 2 diabetes most because restricting carbs reduces the abnormal buildup of insulin levels. This in turn reduces inflammation and improves insulin sensitivity (the body starts using insulin properly—to usher glucose into cells).

A 2005 study published in *Nutrition & Metabolism* found that the keto diet can improve A1C hemoglobin, which gives an overall picture of average blood-sugar levels and is used to diagnose type 2 diabetes. In some patients, a keto diet has even reversed type 2 diabetes.

IMPROVE YOUR GUT HEALTH

You don't eat processed foods or sugars on the Keto Comfort Food Diet—and this is good for your gut. Those foods mess with your gut's "good" bacteria levels, inviting disease as well as gas and bloating. With my diet, you'll be eating foods needed for healthy digestion—high-fiber vegetables, nuts, seeds, and some fruits. You can even eat yogurt and kefir—two foods that supply probiotics (healthy gut bacteria).

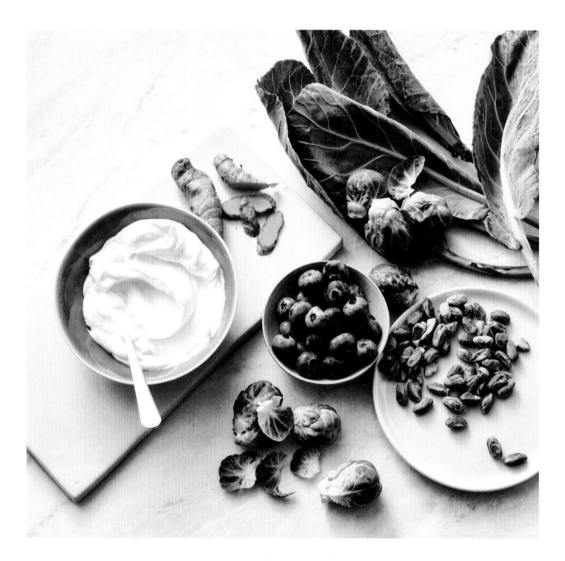

PREVENT BRAIN DISEASES

Neurological diseases such as Alzheimer's are fairly complicated in terms of how and why they develop. What is known, however, is that inflammation, diabetes, high cholesterol, and other diseases are all major risk factors for them. The main reason has to do with the association between diabetes and blood-sugar problems and mental decline. Some medical experts have even renamed Alzheimer's type 3 diabetes because of this association.

Nutritional scientists and brain researchers are now saying that keto can help with several neurological diseases from Alzheimer's to Parkinson's to traumatic brain injuries. It works by helping to preserve and protect the nervous system and cognitive functions. Plus, the keto diet eliminates inflammatory foods (like grains) and reduces sugar intake, both of which are harmful to the brain and particularly detrimental for people with existing neurological conditions.

Of course, the keto diet has long been used in the treatment of epilepsy. Ketone bodies have anticonvulsant properties and thus the ability to control seizures. The reason for this is that the keto diet forces the brain to use ketone bodies instead of glucose for energy, and this reduces the incidence of seizures in many patients, including children.

Please know, too, that high-carb diets can give you brain fog and unclear thinking. But keto dieting increases brain functions such as memory recall and sharp thinking.

ASSIST IN CANCER TREATMENT

At present, researchers are looking into keto diets as a way to support conventional cancer treatments such as radiation and chemotherapy. Ketone bodies are toxic to cancer cells since these runaway cells thrive on glucose. By forcing cancer cells to rely on fat for energy (rather than on sugar), those cells get stressed, weaken, and possibly die off, while normal cells thrive because they can be energized by ketone bodies. This potentially helps improve the response to cancer treatment.

In a 2017 study published in *Current Medicinal Chemistry*, the researchers noted: "The rationale of KD [ketogenic diet] is valid both because it lowers carbohydrate uptake possibly leading to cancer cell starvation and apoptosis [cell death] and, at the same time, increases the levels of ketone bodies available for energy production in normal cells but not in cancer cells."

Pretty impressive, I'd say. Of course, much more research is needed, but the work done thus far appears promising.

ARE YOU IN KETOSIS?

Knowing whether you're in ketosis is important to success on the Keto Comfort Food Diet. For perspective, there are three different types of ketone bodies: beta-hydroxybutyrate, found in the blood; acetoacetate, found in the urine; and acetone, found in your breath. Beta-hydroxybutyrate and acetoacetate are the most abundant and the most involved in fueling the body. Beta-hydroxybutyrate is also what the brain uses for energy. Acetone is the least prevalent and plays the smallest role.

Don't worry about memorizing these chemical names; just know that all three can be measured to determine if you're in ketosis—in other words, is your body burning fat?

Here are some of the tests you can do yourself right at home.

BLOOD TEST

Blood testing is considered to be the number one, most accurate method of measuring levels of ketone bodies in your system. You need a machine and strips for this type of measuring—which makes it the most expensive option compared with the other forms of testing. It involves a finger prick. A good choice is the Precision Xtra with ketone strips, which you can purchase on Amazon.

BREATH TEST

A breath test for ketone bodies detects and measures acetone, which can be smelled on the breath of those in nutritional ketosis. This method of measuring ketone bodies is noninvasive and fairly accurate. The only downside is that it's not as accurate as blood-measuring devices. A breath-measuring device called Ketonix is required.

URINE TEST

Urine readings for levels of ketone bodies are by far the cheapest option available. The urine strips work by detecting compounds excreted by the kidneys. Test strips are available in pharmacies and online.

Typically, you pass the test strip under your urine stream. In about 15 seconds, the tip will turn a shade of pinkish-brown. Match the tip to color codes on the test strip container, and you'll see what state of ketosis you're in—a strong state, a moderate state, a light state, a very light state, or no ketosis at all. It's typically best to be in a moderate or light state. I recommend this method to monitor whether or not you are in ketosis.

WHAT IF YOU'RE NOT IN KETOSIS?

Okay, suppose that testing reveals you're not in ketosis. What should you do?

☐ **CURB YOUR CARBS EVEN MORE.** If you're eating 30 grams daily, you might have to take that down to 20 grams daily.

☐ **SUPPLEMENT WITH MEDIUM-CHAIN TRIGLYCERIDE (MCT) OIL IN YOUR DIET.** Derived from coconut, MCT oil raises ketone bodies in your blood. I talk more about this oil on page 54.

☐ **LOOK INTO TAKING "EXOGENOUS KETONE BODIES."** These powdered supplements are in the form of the ketone body beta-hydroxybutyrate, which your body normally makes on its own. ("Exogenous" means created externally.) The purpose of these supplements is to rapidly restore ketone bodies in your system after a slip of eating too many carbs, as well as to speed up the ketosis process. They are not meant to be used every time you overeat carbs or as an excuse to splurge on carbs. Exogenous ketone bodies do *not* burn fat.

Nonetheless, promising research is emerging on these supplements. A study published in the February 2018 issue of *Obesity* hinted that exogenous ketone bodies reduce hunger hormones and suppress the appetite. This can support weight loss, because if you aren't hungry, you probably aren't going to eat much, or overeat. Another study published in April 2018 in the *Journal of Physiology* noted that these supplements may lower blood sugar.

A downside of these supplements is that they don't taste great and may cause stomach upset. Plus, they're expensive.

Keep in mind, these supplements are not fat-burners. They just support ketosis—the driving factor behind fat-burning. But I do recommend them as insurance for staying in ketosis, as long as you're following my keto dieting recommendations.

☐ **INCREASE YOUR EXERCISE.** Working out empties your body of its glycogen stores. Normally, these are restocked after you eat carbs, which are broken down into glucose and then converted to glycogen. However, because you're minimizing carbs, glycogen stores stay low. In response, your liver increases its production of ketone bodies, which can be used as an alternate fuel source for your muscles.

☐ RAMP UP YOUR FAT INTAKE. You might not be eating enough fat. Remember, consuming fat boosts your ketone levels and helps you reach ketosis. Try eating more good fats such as olive oil, avocado oil, coconut oil, or butter.

☐ WATCH YOUR PROTEIN INTAKE. Excessive protein may suppress ketone body production, so don't go overboard on this macronutrient.

You can easily come out of ketosis without knowing it if you stop tracking your ketone body levels. If you find yourself not losing weight, it probably means that you are not truly on keto or in ketosis. Keep testing and keep making adjustments to your diet and exercise program! When you discover through testing that you're in ketosis, this confirmation is very motivating to stay with the plan.

HOW FAST WILL I LOSE WEIGHT?

Attention, please: How fast can you expect to see results once you start the Keto Comfort Food Diet?

It's hard to give an exact answer because everyone is different. If you have a lot of weight to lose, for example, you'll likely experience faster weight loss in the beginning. What's more, your body needs time to become fat-adapted. For instance, if you're coming off a typical junk-food, processed-food diet, and your body has never been powered by ketone bodies before, your fat-adaptation period might take a little longer—anywhere between 1 and 2 weeks.

That said, based on what I observed in my test group, the average weight loss on this diet plays out like this.

FIRST 3 DAYS. On my Keto Cleanse, expect to *possibly* lose more than 1 pound a day. This rate of weight loss is what I observed in my test group.

WEEK 1. During week 1, expect to see a rapid drop in pounds—anywhere from 3 pounds to as much as 10 pounds, especially if you follow the accelerated tier. This is what I observed in my own test group, and it supports the evidence seen in studies of weight loss on ketogenic diets.

Chalk this up to the fact that keto dieting releases a lot of water weight. However, this water loss may also result in dehydration and constipation, so swill down more H_2O than normal to keep your digestion train on track. But you will also be losing pure fat along with water, and you'll quickly see and feel your body shrinking. You might even be slipping into a smaller size by the weekend.

WEEK 2 AND BEYOND. You'll lose 2 to 5 pounds a week. At this point, you're becoming "fat-adapted"; your body is switching from burning carbs to burning fat. This rate of weight loss is consistent with research. One study found that obese patients shed 30 pounds after 2 months on a keto diet. That's nearly 4 pounds a week!

LONGER-TERM. As you approach your ideal weight and have gone beyond the initial 21 days and moved on to the Basic Keto Comfort Food Diet, your weight loss might slow down a bit. This is normal.

You might have a few weeks where it seems like you aren't losing an ounce; don't be discouraged. It's just your body readjusting. Weigh yourself a week or two later and you'll be down a few more pounds. People on my diet stay with the plan—without discouragement or deprivation—because the comfort foods I provide make it easier to follow.

MAINTENANCE. After you reach your ideal weight on the Keto Comfort Food Diet, you'll switch over to Keto Comfort Phasing, which is more liberal and introduces more foods. This is a plan you can use for the rest of your life to stay lean, fit, and healthy.

The key is to stay the course, celebrate how good you feel, and keep testing to make sure you're still in ketosis.

The Keto Comfort Food Diet puts your body into the happiest condition you can be in as a dieter. Not only does it burn fat rapidly and improve lots of health parameters, it requires no grit-your-teeth-and-do-it willpower, no hunger, no cravings, and no dietary misery of any kind. After a week or so, you'll feel better, lighter, and more energetic and focused than you've felt in years.

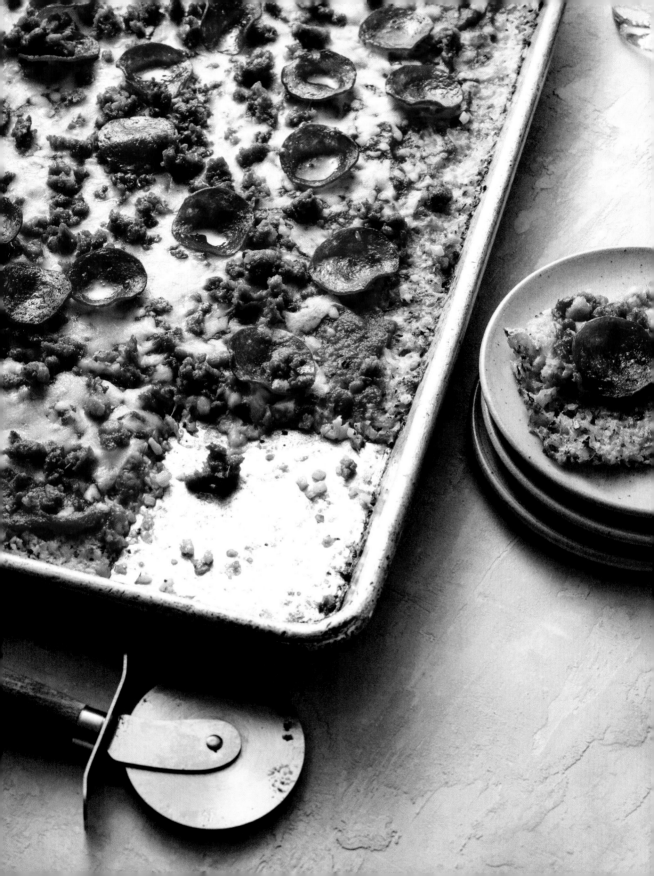

THE KETO DIETER'S MISSING LINK

Yes, you burn fat at an astounding rate on a keto diet and get healthier. But remember the problem I described in the introduction: For the most part, the meals on keto diets can be boring and pretty bland—which is why a lot of dieters can't stick to these plans for very long. The problem is that keto diets lack the "comfort factor."

By that, I mean the element of food that gives it an emotional lift when you eat it. You know, like the favorite foods of your childhood, or meals linked to a person, place, or time with which the food has a positive association. For example, for me, eating red-sauced pasta and my mother's meatballs evokes pleasant memories of my youth in suburban Queens.

Comfort foods are also typically calorie-dense, rich, and sweet. Think ice cream, French fries, fried chicken, mac and cheese, a big bowl of pasta, or a hunk of crusty white bread with a creamy soup. The comfort factor is the hallmark of truly delicious cooking.

So this missing *comfort factor* is something that I and others don't like about typical keto diets. No one wants to eat tasteless food on a diet. It won't help you stay on a plan, lose weight, or even keep it off. If I believed that for the rest of my life I couldn't enjoy an ice cream sundae, I'd probably just throw away my scale and let the nuts and sprinkles fall where they may.

I got pretty serious and pretty determined about solving this problem and transforming keto foods into keto *comfort* foods. All my nutritional and culinary experience told me that I could do it—so driven partly by gut feel, I started experimenting. When it came to keto foods, I became more of a "reinventor" than an inventor in my "lab," better known as my kitchen.

Eventually, I found that I could modify my favorite foods and turn them into keto foods—without the carbs and sugar—all delicious and mouthwatering. I could take my favorite comfort foods and transform them into dishes that would trigger weight loss, burn fat, and promote all the health benefits related to keto diets. And thus, the Keto Comfort Food Diet was born.

MY ADVENTURES WITH FLAVOR

My main focus was on flavor, something I grew up with as an Italian-American with a mom and grandmother who instinctively, using their taste buds, cooked with bold, lusty flavors.

Much of what I learned about cooking came from spending time with them in their kitchens. They based their recipes (unwritten!) on a template of aromas and tastes, which they adjusted to bring out the flavors of the main ingredients in a dish. For example, for my mother's meatballs (the best in the world), she would start by pureeing garlic and onions in a blender with chicken stock, then combine that mixture with meat, bread crumbs, eggs, Parmigiano-Reggiano, red pepper flakes for heat, and salt—all formed into balls. Then she'd sauté them in olive oil and dunk them in marinara sauce at the end. Oh—and her marinara sauce? Her secret to boosting its flavor was to splash in a bit of balsamic vinegar. I noticed these simple habits when I was a kid, and they have helped me in my adult life to become a better chef.

But not every culinary influence was Italian. My home when I was growing up was within a neighborhood of several dozen ethnicities and restaurants to serve them. So when it came to eating out, we were quite adventuresome. I ate Japanese food, Cantonese, Mexican, Indian, and others. Trips to these eateries were like free trips to other countries. What could be more fun than that? For me discovering new flavors has been a part of my life—then and now. The way flavors work together in a dish is sheer magic, moving a dish from boring to beautiful. Flavor brings food—including keto food—to life.

Technically, flavor is a good balance of the five fundamental factors in food—salty (Parmesan, capers, and salt), sweet (berries, cinnamon, and coconut), sour (vinegar, lemons, and limes), bitter (mustard, coffee, and Swiss chard), and umami (mushrooms, meat, and tomatoes). In Asian cultures, when these flavors are in balance, the body is also considered in tune. I've adopted this philosophy. Good food with balanced flavors is essential to the body's well-being.

I put this philosophy into practice with my keto comfort food recipes. I wanted them to be vibrant and energizing, with the ability to register a series of bright notes with each bite, each note clear on its own, and all in perfect harmony. Of course, you'll have to be the judge as you sample each recipe and pick your favorites.

Every recipe in this book went through several drafts before making the final cut. I retool and rework a dish until I nail it.

I like to play with the tension among different flavors. Sometimes unlikely ingredients seem like strange bedfellows, but often they come together seamlessly to create something delicious. For example, did you know that adding a bit of salt to something sweet can make it sweeter? Salt makes everything brighter and stronger, without tasting salty. Just a little pinch completely transforms a dish. Parmesan cheese, capers, and other condiments are also good ways to add salt.

Or how about putting coffee into chocolate (permissible in small amounts on my diet)? It can accent the chocolaty flavor and make it bolder. Dull food can be saved!

In addition, I tested each dish by finishing the entire meal, since a dish can taste quite different at bite two than at bite twenty. (You can understand why it's easy for a restaurant chef who's in charge of creating new menu items to gain weight!)

When transforming familiar comfort foods into keto comfort foods, I looked exclusively to my palate for approval. Keto comfort foods simply had to taste as good as, if not better than, their nondiet counterparts.

For the Keto Comfort Food Diet and its recipes, I invented dishes according to specific checkpoints: no starchy carbs, abundant in fat, deliciously seasoned proteins, and sweets without sugar—in short, gorgeous plates of keto food. A tall order for sure.

FAREWELL, MY LOVELY STARCHES

Replacing starchy carbs was the biggest challenge. I began to experiment with as many alternatives and swaps as I could think of. It all started with vegetables. . . .

Cauliflower is a good example. Once upon a time, it was not the most popular veggie on the produce block. But like a wallflower who blossoms into the most beautiful girl in school, so goes cauliflower. We now have so many more ideas for what to do with it in addition to drenching it in cheese sauce. Cauliflower, for instance, is the new pizza crust.

As for me, I found additional ways to make riced cauliflower taste better than regular rice, and mashed cauliflower better than mashed potatoes.

I have long used spaghetti squash or "zoodles"—strands of zucchini that look like spaghetti—as substitutes for pasta, but I wanted to discover other vegetables that could replace starchy comfort foods.

I started using portobello mushrooms for hamburger buns; eggplant slices for manicotti, lasagna noodles, and rollatini; and butternut squash sliced into fettuccine noodles. The results are amazing. In natural foods stores and in some supermarkets, you can find many veggies already spiralized into noodles and packaged.

As an advocate of plant-based eating, I love the fact that substituting vegetables for pasta and other starchy carbs means fewer carbs, fewer processed ingredients, no gluten, more fiber, and of course, all the wonderful color and interesting flavor variations!

For desserts such as cakes, cookies, brownies, and so on, I tested ingredients outside of the sphere of flour. Almond flour (finely ground almonds) can be substituted for wheat flour in cakes, cookies, brownie bars, and pancakes. Almond flour can also be used as a coating for protein entrées such as sautéed fish fillets and chicken cutlets.

Almond flour is low in carbs, about 24 grams per cup, as opposed to wheat flour, which has about 95 grams per cup. And eating almonds every day carries broad health benefits that will do just about everything for you except your laundry.

Another great flour fill-in is coconut flour. I love working with it because it gives a moist consistency to baked goods.

What's more, finely ground flaxseeds can be added to these flours for extra protein, healthy fats, and disease-preventing compounds.

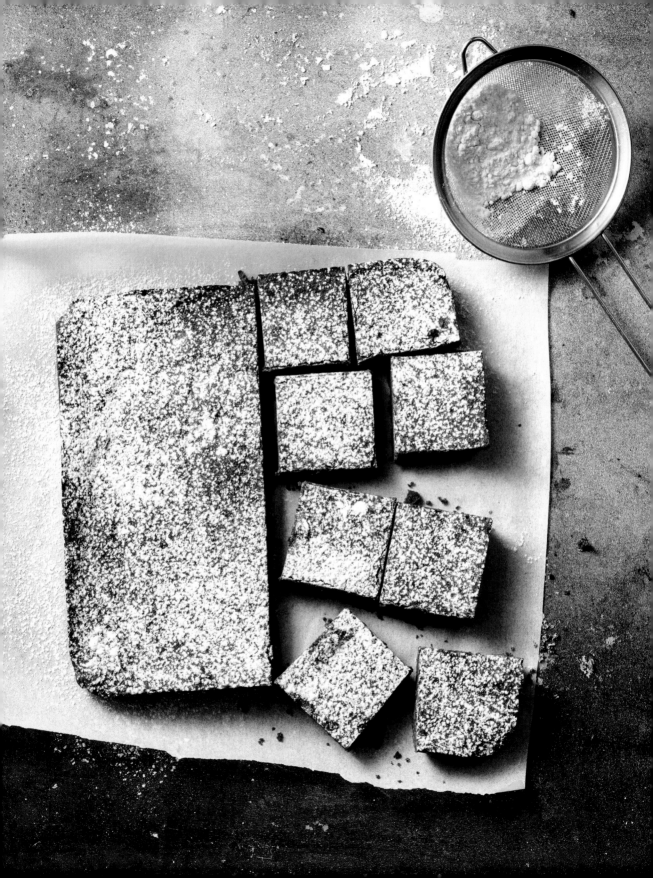

SWEET RELEASE

One big reason I like ketogenic nutrition is that it treats your addiction to something that's pure, white, and deadly. Sounds like a drug? It is. It's sugar!

Sugar addiction is a problem. Some experts say that it's the hardest addiction to kick, perhaps six to eight times harder than quitting cocaine. One downside to sugar is that it imparts a "natural high" by triggering the brain to pump out the feel-good chemical serotonin. You want that feeling, so you eat more sugar. Here's an interesting study from Yale University: When shown photographs of a milkshake made with chocolate ice cream, women displayed brain activity on a par with that of addicts who craved drugs or alcohol.

If you feel like you're hooked on sugar, I get it. I've never met a cheesecake I didn't like. For years, I'd finish off a meal with some kind of sweet dessert and lick my fingers every time I frosted a cake. I tried to curb my sweet tooth, but being in the restaurant business made it tough, because part of my job was to concoct desserts of all kinds. Eating a little too much sugar didn't help my weight much either.

So my next biggest challenge was sugar replacement. A keto diet simply cannot have even a smidgeon of sugar, or else you'll be booted out of ketosis, and your weight loss will slow to a crawl. For years, I've explored the use of natural sugar substitutes. Not chemical-laden artificial sweeteners, but the newer crop of more natural alternatives on the market, such as stevia (which is calorie-free) and monk fruit—all of which work beautifully on my Keto Comfort Food Diet.

Once I discovered keto dieting and got off sugar, I couldn't believe how fast my sweet cravings vanished. I was eating more protein and fat—two very satiating macronutrients that stayed in my stomach longer and didn't release energy as fast as sugar. The veggies in my keto diet worked for the same reason: They slowed down the release of energy from food. Also, rather than start off the day with my usual bagel (the kind of breakfast that ignites sugar cravings later), I'd have a protein-rich keto breakfast of eggs and breakfast meat—both of which annihilated sweet cravings.

Once you kick sugar, you'll be doing your body a world of good. Just 1 teaspoon of sugar lowers the function of the liver by 50 percent for up to 6 hours. Sugar is not great for your skin, either. It promotes bacterial growth, making it more acne prone. It's also part of a process that produces advanced glycation end products (AGEs), which accelerate aging and cause skin wrinkles. And then there's the damage done to teeth. When we started feeding people more and more sugar and easily digestible carbohydrates, that is when chronic diseases started.

Trust me, once you go keto, you'll enjoy much better health. If you do want something sweet, I've created a host of keto comfort food treats that are sugar-free and won't reawaken that sweet desire.

HELLO FAT!

In several of my past books, I had worked hard at reducing the fat in recipes. But with keto recipes, I had to work hard at upping the fat! I didn't have to swap out fat with alternatives such as cornstarch or yogurt; I could use the real deal. This was liberating, because as chefs, we use all sorts of fats—butter, cream, lard, goose fat, and more—to carry flavor and impart a rich mouthfeel to dishes.

PUNCHING UP PROTEIN

Nothing kills a commitment to healthy eating faster than boredom. To further battle keto meal monotony, I had to perform some spectacular feats with protein. After all, who can subsist on baked skinless chicken breasts, the ubiquitous base upon which many weight-loss diets are built? I mean, how many times have you found yourself craving a naked, unseasoned piece of chicken? Not me, I'd throw up the white flag and order KFC if the road to lasting weight loss looked like an endless parade of plain chicken breasts.

I figured out some ways to break the monotony of not only chicken but other proteins, too: turkey, fish, and beef among them. Nonetheless, let me start with chicken. I've made my own luscious keto version of fried chicken, submerging thighs in a foamy egg bath and then dredging them in a spicy almond flour. Because oil is not off limits on keto, I then simply fry them up and I have moist, crunchy Hot Crispy Keto Fried Chicken (page 221)—my version of KFC!—to enjoy.

I don't eat as much beef as I used to, but taking beef away from me entirely would make me quite depressed. Yes, I know that the antimeat cops have declared that one person's steak has become every person's poison.

On the Keto Comfort Food Diet, if you want beef, go ahead and enjoy it. It helps create stronger muscles, builds better bones, boosts the growth of brain cells, and combats sexual dysfunction. Beef has no equal as a protein source, and has an amino-acid profile that's second to none.

Then there's fish—something most people are afraid to cook for fear of screwing it up. I've got a few tricks up my sleeve, though, that will have you cooking all types of fish like a pro. The great thing about preparing fish for a keto diet is that you can cook it in butter—which is really ideal for seafood. I love to sear fish in butter until it has a nice golden crust, then finish cooking it in the oven to keep the fish moist and flaky—heavenly. My favorite fish spice is Cajun (check out my Cajun Fish "Tacos" on page 198); of course, simple salt, pepper, and some white wine to pump up flavor, too. Like your fish fried? Wait until you try my seasoned nut crust on your fish. So don't discount fish. It is easy and quick to cook, plus it provides essential fatty acids that can't be made by the body.

Chicken—white and dark meat—is a great protein for getting rid of excess body fat. It contains less fat and cholesterol than many other animal proteins. It is also a cornucopia of vitamins and minerals, including niacin, vitamins B_6 and B_{12}, iron, selenium, and zinc.

I like to stretch my proteins, too—a habit I picked up from the cooks in my family. They'd make sensational soup that began with a chicken or beef stock, which had at its core the carcass, leftover meat, and skin from a whole roasted chicken. The already browned skin contributed both color and flavor to the stock. Watching my mother and grandmother taught me one more rather unbelievable secret to great stock: vinegar. They'd add a tablespoon of cider vinegar to their stock at the beginning of cooking. As the stock simmers, the vinegar does something amazing: It helps the bones give up their protein to the stock, making it healthier and much more flavorful.

I tried this secret with a creamy keto comfort soup. I kept tasting and tasting it. It didn't need more salt or pepper. But it was still flat. I remembered the vinegar trick. I stirred in some apple cider vinegar. Voilà! It amped up the flavor like crazy.

When you incorporate some of these techniques into your cooking, you won't feel like you're missing anything.

A couple of important tips about protein:

☐ When possible, purchase only organic, grass-fed, and/or pasture-raised meat, poultry, and eggs.

☐ Choose only cuts labeled "no antibiotics added" or "certified organic."

☐ Go for wild-caught fish over farmed fish (which tends to have a spongy texture and a bland flavor). Watch out for farmed shrimp, too. It's treated intensively with antibiotics and can have high levels of contaminants. A good website to consult as you make seafood choices is seafoodwatch.org.

DISCOVER THE KETO COMFORT DIFFERENCE

Try as many recipes as possible from this book. I mean, who can resist food like lasagna, fried chicken, burgers, fries, chocolate chip peanut butter cookies, cheesecake, or ice cream? These are all keto and they are all here—they're just keto versions of what you love to eat. With these recipes, everything about keto has changed. Now, you can make these incredible, creative keto recipes—and you'll never look back.

Once you get the hang of all this goodness, be creative and experiment. I love to go to different markets and wander around the food aisles with nothing specific in mind. I just see what pops into my imagination. One time, I went out and bought a bunch of vegetables and herbs and asked myself "What can I make with these?" Back in my kitchen, I had a ball. I came up with mustard greens sautéed with bacon, garlic, and ginger; pureed cauliflower with parsley, thyme, and butter; and a salad of radishes with dried cranberries and goat cheese. Here were three amazing dishes, each one a delicious keto side dish. It's just about experimenting. There's really no limit to what you can do with a little creativity.

As you can see, doing the Keto Comfort Food Diet does not mean relegating yourself to tasteless dry meat and vegetables with no seasoning. Now you can enjoy flavor-packed food that is low-carb, high-fat, and moderate-protein—prepared creatively and smartly. "Enjoy" is the key word here . . . no longer do you have to feel deprived. You can indulge in your favorite comfort foods—some good old-fashioned happy food—then sit back and get excited by your fast-shrinking waistline.

SECRET KETO COMFORT FOOD INGREDIENTS

From a culinary standpoint, I've always hunted enthusiastically for new ingredients because I'm a naturally curious person who never tires of new experiences. Keto cooking presented lots of new challenges, though I found I could deploy ingredients that I've used in my previous cooking makeovers. But a whole host of keto-friendly ingredients revealed themselves as I began this journey. Below you'll find a rundown of all the key foods that put the "comfort" in keto.

APPLE CIDER VINEGAR

I love all sorts of vinegars and use them frequently in a variety of dishes. But when it comes to a keto diet, apple cider vinegar is my favorite. Fermented from the juice of apples and full of beneficial enzymes, apple cider vinegar supports ketone production in the body and improves ketosis. Some studies suggest that it has a modest fat-burning effect in the body. It also helps in the digestion of fats.

I have also found it extremely helpful on the Keto Comfort Phasing part of the diet when you get to eat more carbs two to three times a week. Here's the deal: Apple cider vinegar is extremely beneficial for improving blood-sugar stability (which can waver when you eat carb-rich meals). In fact, research has shown that apple cider vinegar can reduce the glycemic index of white bread from 100 to 64. This simply means that the vinegar prevents the huge spike in blood sugar that you'd normally get from eating white bread.

AVOCADO

This keto-friendly fruit (yes, it's a fruit) is more than just a component of salads, sandwiches, or guacamole. It is an important keto ingredient that can be used in keto desserts such as pies, mousses, and puddings. In fact, when I made a chocolate avocado pudding and served it to guests, at first they turned their noses up, until several loud yums erupted from those daring enough to sample it.

Because my pudding was a comfort food recipe, I should add that I put a dollop of real whipped cream on top—which is perfectly acceptable in keto dieting! I love avocados not only for their versatility and taste but for their amazing nutrition. They're loaded with healthy fats that honor your body.

BUTTER

Ahh. . . . Before I was into downsizing the calories and fat in recipes, I cooked with a lot of butter. It's gratifying to welcome it back to my kitchen since keto meals allow it. I admit it; I missed butter. Oh, did I miss it. Nothing washes over veggies or tastes quite so delicious in cookies like melted butter.

A tip: I prefer to use unsalted butter because I don't want to risk oversalting a dish. Salt is a preservative; it increases the shelf life of butter. Unsalted is fresher and tastes sweeter. When shopping for butter, look for products that are produced from all grass-fed cow's milk and certified organic.

Feel free to use ghee, too, a form of butter that's supposed to be almost miraculously healthy. Ghee is the result of simmering butter over medium heat and skimming off the milk solids that float to the top. This method turns solid, perishable butter into a shelf-stable semiliquid. It's safe for lactose-intolerant people because the milk proteins have been removed.

The first time I tasted ghee, I was wowed. Its buttery flavor exploded on my tongue. "Now that's what butter should taste like!" I shouted. I started ticking off all the ways I could add ghee to keto recipes: in fudge, brownies, cakes, sauces, sautéing, and pureed veggies. You can safely sauté with ghee, too, because it has a very high smoke point (485°F—olive oil's smoke point is 405°F; unclarified butter's is 350°F).

CELTIC SEA SALT

Speaking of salt, it happens to be quite important on a keto diet—advice you don't usually hear. After you've been on the Keto Comfort Food Diet for a while, your insulin sensitivity will improve—a sign that your insulin levels have fallen. When this happens, the kidneys churn out excess fluid—which means you'll be in the bathroom more often. This will subside eventually, but while it's happening, you'll lose some electrolytes, and salt is one.

Remember that the loss of electrolytes can increase your risk of temporarily experiencing keto flu. You can lose electrolytes because you're drinking—and excreting—more water. So you need to ensure that you're replenishing your body's electrolytes, and one of the easiest ways to do that is to get salt (sodium) into your system. I certainly have no problem adding salt to any foods that can use some extra seasoning! Also, make sure you're eating your nonstarchy veggies, because they're high in electrolytes, too.

What kind of salt is best? I like Celtic sea salt. It is the least processed and has the fewest chemicals of all salts, and retains as many as 84 minerals that were originally in the sea. You can buy Celtic sea salt in health food stores and natural foods stores.

CHOCOLATE

Yes, chocolate is keto-friendly—with a few caveats. It's got to be sugar-free. For example, I love stevia-sweetened chocolate baking chips as a swap for regular chocolate chips, such as Lily's brand Dark Chocolate Premium Baking Chips. They supply zero sugar and fewer calories per ounce than regular chocolate chips. This product also contains about 1 gram more fat than regular chocolate chips—which is great for keto diets (the more fat the better).

I also use unsweetened cocoa powder in recipes. It is rich in flavonoids—beneficial dietary antioxidants that protect the body from heart disease, diabetes, and cancer, and are also abundant in fruits, vegetables, and wine. Good deal!

CITRUS

In my world, there are three basic spices: salt, pepper, and citrus juice. Because keto diets limit fruit, that leaves lemon and lime juice, but that's okay. There's something about citrus that not only brightens and enlivens a dish but also primes the other ingredients. Go for fresh juice, too—not the bottled versions. They give too much of a lemon or lime or preservative taste—and nothing else. This throws the whole dish off.

COCONUT AMINOS

Coconut aminos is a liquid condiment that is great if you're allergic to soy and gluten. Available at organic and natural foods grocery stores and many conventional supermarkets, it is made from organic coconut sap, which is loaded with minerals, vitamin C, B vitamins, and amino acids. As such, coconut aminos have a higher amino acid content than soy-based sauces.

I use coconut aminos to replace soy sauce and Worcestershire sauce in recipes, and you can do the same. It imparts a delicious, deep, salty soy sauce flavor, and makes a terrific taste booster.

CONDIMENTS AND SAUCES

Remember how I keep harping on the fact that typical keto diets are blah? I combat "keto blah" by using lots of different condiments, which are useful when you're cooking up something keto very quickly (without any recipe). Unfortunately, a lot of condiments contain added sugars and carbs and can be detrimental to ketosis. But there are also plenty of sugar-free condiments that are safe to use and that I recommend:

Anchovy paste	*Fish sauce*	*Hot sauce*	*Salsa (sugar-free)*
Clam juice	*Horseradish*	*Mustard*	

CREAM

Here is a luscious dairy food you can use wantonly in keto cooking—in soups, sauces, purees, baked goods, and more. In French and other dairy-loving cuisines, it's depended on as a thickener to provide smooth texture and rich mouthfeel—and it does the same for keto comfort food recipes.

EXTRACTS

These are miracle workers—concentrated flavor bombs, all without carbs, that I drop in various dishes to bring out their best. I use extracts like crazy in keto cooking and baking. I'm talking about not only the usual suspects like vanilla and almond extracts but also peppermint, maple, chocolate, and more. They are made from essential oils found in certain plant foods. The oils are then distilled to produce pure extracts. A scant teaspoon or less is all you need to flavor desserts, cakes, cookies, and other recipes.

EXTRA-VIRGIN OLIVE OIL

I prefer extra-virgin olive oil to regular olive oil because there is a real taste difference between the two. For background, extra-virgin means the oil is the product of the very first pressing of the olives; it simply tastes better than any subsequent pressing, which will contain far less olive taste and more of the bitter pomace taste of the olive pit and skins. That bitter taste is oleic acid, released as the olive oil is broken down by the pressing. In keto cooking, extra-virgin olive oil makes all the difference.

FLOURS (LOW-CARB)

Traditional flours like white flour and whole wheat flour—any high-carb flour, really—are avoided in keto cooking. Fortunately, as I mentioned earlier, there are amazing swaps that work just as well, but without all the carbs. Here are my favorites.

ALMOND FLOUR. Made of very finely ground blanched almonds, almond flour adds flavor and texture to cakes and confections.

COCONUT FLOUR. This flour comes from coconut meat. Most of the oil has been squeezed out to produce coconut oil; the remaining material is ground into a powder. Its consistency resembles that of wheat flour, but coconut flour is higher in fiber and protein than wheat flour.

PSYLLIUM. High in fiber, this seed is used in some bulk-forming natural laxatives and in some breakfast cereals. In baking, it adds volume and helps the ingredients bind together. There is strong evidence that psyllium fiber curbs hunger to help with weight loss and prevent obesity. Use psyllium husk powder as a low-carb, low-glycemic substitute for all or some of the flour in recipes.

SUNFLOWER SEED MEAL AND PUMPKIN SEED FLOUR. If you're allergic to almond flour or coconut flour, these are good options. Ground from seeds, these flours are high in fiber and vitamins and minerals such as vitamin E, B vitamins, copper, selenium, and phosphorus. They combine well with other low-carb flours in recipes. You can make your own seed flours using a food processor or spice grinder.

HERBS AND SPICES

A lot of seasonings contain added sugar and carbs—and therefore aren't keto-friendly. For this reason, you want to make friends with certain herbs and spices. They are more than just flavoring agents; they are also packed with phytochemicals that have disease-fighting power. In addition to salt, pepper, and citrus, some of the best herbs and spices to use include:

Basil	*Cinnamon*	*Ginger*	*Rosemary*
Cardamom	*Cumin*	*Nutmeg*	*Thyme*
Cayenne pepper	*Curry powder*	*Oregano*	*Turmeric*
Chili powder	*Dill*	*Parsley*	
Cilantro	*Garlic*	*Red pepper flakes*	

MCT OIL

I love MCT oil, otherwise known as medium-chain triglyceride oil. It's practically a keto staple, since it's the easiest fat to convert into ketone bodies for energy and fat-burning. Plus, it is thermogenic (meaning it raises the body's temperature to burn calories faster), boosts the metabolism, and prevents the accumulation of fat. It can even trigger weight loss and help melt away a muffin top or unwanted belly fat.

Most oils are constructed entirely of long-chain triglycerides, or LCTs, which are more than 12 carbons long. Medium-chain triglycerides are 6 to 12 carbons long. The distinction matters because our bodies metabolize MCTs differently than they do LCTs. MCTs head directly from the intestinal tract to the liver, where they're promptly burned off as fuel. That means less is available to be circulated throughout the body and deposited in fat tissue.

MCT oil is made from coconut oil (which is another good keto oil), but there are differences. For one thing, coconut oil is not 100 percent MCTs. Coconut oil contains various fatty acids, around 60 percent of which fit the chemical classification of MCTs. Plus, not all of these fatty acids help burn fat.

When you use pure MCT oil, you're getting 100 percent MCTs. Among these, the most superior is C8, caprylic acid. It has the most superior ketone body–producing profile. When you purchase MCT oil, make sure it is formulated mostly with C8. MCT oil is generally found in the supplement section of the grocery store.

MCT oil has a light, neutral flavor. Try it as a salad dressing with a little vinegar, herbs, and spices; add it to smoothies and drizzle it over vegetables.

PARMESAN "CRISPS"

These are crunchy snacks made from 100 percent Parmesan cheese. They make great cracker-like snacks for dipping and replacing croutons in salads, among other uses. The product trade name for these delights is Whisps.

I like to use them as a swap for bread crumbs in one of my favorite foods—meatloaf. I simply crumble the crisps, and they serve as a flavorful bulking and moistening agent. I know what you're thinking: "This is meatloaf, buddy! How dare you mess with it!"

You've got to mess with meatloaf when you're converting it to a keto version. With the crisps, you'll end up with a full-flavored and meaty meatloaf that tastes substantial, a savory classic dish so good that it might even taste like the one your mom or grandma used to make.

Parmesan crisps are also great for making delicious, keto-friendly meatballs.

PROTEIN POWDERS

Protein powders are typically ingredients added to smoothies and shakes as a way to get a concentrated infusion of nutrients that will help accelerate your metabolism. It is well known that protein boosts your fat-burning and enhances satiety.

But another way to use these products is in baking to make cake-like and bread-like items without the carbs, which will kick you out of ketosis.

There seem to be a zillion protein powders on the market, so which one is best for a keto diet? Look for one that is 100 percent whey protein isolate, zero carb, and gluten-, lactose-, and aspartame-free. Each scoop should have around 2 grams of protein, a little fat, and zero carbs. Read labels to make sure.

SHIRATAKI NOODLES

When you're not using zoodles or butternut fettuccine as stand-ins for pasta, try shirataki noodles. They're made from yam flour (konjac) or tofu and they have virtually no carbs. Don't worry; they don't taste like tofu, but have the flavor of light egg noodles. They come in three shapes—spaghetti, fettuccine, and angel hair. There is also a similar rice-like product made with yam flour with no carbs, gluten, or preservatives, and practically no calories. Check out the website, miraclenoodle.com.

SWEETENERS

When it comes to sweetening foods on a keto diet, sugar and its cousins like honey, maple syrup, agave syrup, and molasses will definitely be MIA. But that's okay—for two reasons. One is health-related. As I've mentioned, excess sugar is one of the dietary causes of cardiovascular diseases, fatty liver, type 2 diabetes, obesity, and more. Second, eating sugar kicks you out of ketosis fast.

Fortunately, there are other sweeteners you can use instead. The best are stevia and erythritol. For stevia, I prefer the Sweet Leaf product. This is a 100 percent natural sugar substitute made from stevia, a carb-free, calorie-free herb said to be three hundred times sweeter than sugar. Stevia is natural in the sense that it is not a chemical concocted in a lab; it's a natural extract from the stevia plant. It doesn't raise blood sugar. It's filled with antioxidants, and it might even cut your cravings for sweets.

Erythritol is a sugar alcohol derived from corn. It is an excellent sweetener in keto cooking. It contains no artificial ingredients, preservatives, or flavorings. It's zero-calorie, nonglycemic, and has no effect on blood glucose or insulin levels. Nor does it have a weird aftertaste. It measures just like sugar in recipes and is the only sugar replacement I know of that caramelizes like real sugar. I use regular erythritol, brown sugar erythritol, and confectioners' erythritol in my recipes.

Please stay away from artificial sweeteners like Splenda, sucralose, and aspartame, although they, too, are carb- and calorie-free. You can get hit with blood-sugar spikes and cravings from ingesting these fake sweeteners. They can also halt ketosis and interfere with hormones that affect weight.

XANTHAN GUM

Xanthan gum is a natural food additive that's commonly added to foods as a thickener or stabilizer; it adds volume and viscosity to baked goods. A strong versatile ingredient that can instantly thicken just about anything, it has a pleasant mouthfeel that will be perceived as fatty, although no fat is there. Use xanthan gum in baking to replace gluten.

These keto-friendly ingredients are examples of how, with a little ingenuity, your favorite comfort food recipes can be reinvented. Then you can enjoy what you've cooked up, and unlike previous diets you've tried, your delicious, transformed keto diet will last longer than half of Monday.

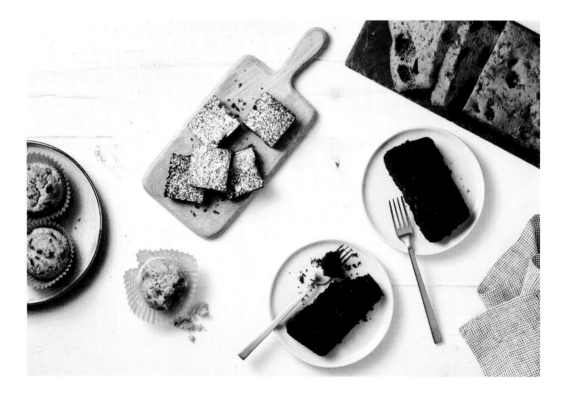

FAT-BURNING FOODS

So you're ready to start my Keto Comfort Food Diet. Now what? What can you eat on this diet?

In two words: real food. But real food, prepared keto comfort food–style!

Real food comes from the ground and is locally sourced, along with properly raised meat, poultry, and fish; it is food without any unnecessary ingredients, the kind of food that doesn't need packages or even labels. So foods like pastas, cereals, wheat-based breads, cookies, dairy products, and soft drinks—items that are typically produced in a factory—are out. Healthy, wholesome fats, vegetables, chicken, beef, and fish are in.

The quality of your food really matters. If possible, it's a smart move to choose meats that are organic, grass-fed, and pasture-raised. The same goes for eggs—from local farmers or pasture-raised hens. Select grass-fed butter and organic dairy foods and vegetables. Trust me, all of this will taste better. After I started cooking with, and eating, organic foods, I couldn't believe their superior flavor.

Eating conventional or nonorganic food won't prevent you from achieving ketosis, but high-quality food, free of toxins, is better for your health in general. Try your best to buy the highest-quality real food whenever you can. Prepared well, real food will always be more palatable, tasty, and full of goodness than highly processed food.

Plus, it's a better source of nutrients on which your body can run efficiently. Your body is like a car. It can run okay as long as it has gas, oil, and tires, but why not try to make it run like a Ferrari? We can all be brighter, stronger, and more productive versions of ourselves by eating better, so why not respect and treat our bodies like the high-performance machines they are.

THE CARB COUNTDOWN

On the Keto Comfort Food Diet, it's important to track your total carbs with a limit of 20 to 40 grams per day, especially if you're new to keto nutrition. Staying at 30 grams daily is ideal.

Not counting carbs is one of the big reasons why some keto dieters don't get the fast results they are expecting. Every now and then, you might go over 40 grams. That's okay—just don't do it too often or get too close to 50 grams daily. The lower your daily carb count, the better it is for fat-burning.

I like to count "total carbs" because they are always reflected on nutritional labeling and in food information. I don't worry about "net carbs," which is a calculation representing the carbs in a food minus the grams of fiber. It is not a legal definition.

Counting total carbs helps keep you in nutritional ketosis so that you're always burning pure fat. By contrast, eating too many grams of carbs will kick you out of ketosis. There are carbs in certain keto foods that you might be unaware of. For example, eating too many nuts can push your daily carb count over 50 grams and thus interfere with ketosis. You can count carbs by consulting a nutrient counter book, a special app, or a tracker like MyFitnessPal. I've included carb counts below for certain foods you'll enjoy on my plan. The recipes also include carb counts.

Now . . . speaking of enjoyment, next up are the "real" ketogenic foods that you'll be eating for success.

KETO COMFORT FATS

Fats and oils form the foundation of the Keto Comfort Food Diet, so you get to eat plenty of these. They help keep your body in ketosis—burning fat for fuel rather than carbs or protein.

While following this diet, it's important to select quality fats—those that are better for you than others. There are three categories of fats from which to choose.

SATURATED FATS

Generally solid at room temperature, saturated fat is good for your health, contrary to popular belief. It has been well researched and found to lower LDL and improve HDL cholesterol—both the bad and good cholesterol indicators—and it also supports your immune system and contributes to the manufacture of hormones.

These good keto sources of saturated fat contain 0.4 to zero carbs.

Grass-fed and organic red meats, poultry dark meat, and eggs

High-fat dairy foods like ghee, grass-fed butter, and heavy cream

Coconut oil

MCT oil

MONOUNSATURATED FATS

Remaining liquid at room temperature, these fats have been shown to help regulate insulin and blood sugar, normalize wayward cholesterol, trim belly fat, and boost heart health.

Good keto sources of monounsaturated fats include:

Avocados (½ cup slices): 6 grams of carbs

Extra-virgin olive oil, avocado oil, and macadamia nut oil: 0 carbs

Nuts, nut butters, seeds, and seed butters: See the charts on pages 62 and 64 for carb counts

OMEGA-3 FATS

These special fats boost metabolism, burn fat, and help improve transmission of mood-regulating brain chemicals. Omega-3 fats also increase oxygenation of the blood, which means better delivery of nutrients to your muscles for growth and repair after exercising.

Sources of omega-3 fats include:

Fatty fish like trout, mackerel, salmon, and tuna: 0 carbs

Nuts and seeds like almonds, walnuts, pecans, Brazil nuts, flaxseeds, chia seeds, hemp seeds, sunflower seeds, and pumpkin seeds: See the charts for nuts and seeds on pages 62 and 64 for carb counts

Flaxseed oil, sesame oil, fish oil, and avocado oil: 0 carbs

Eat a variety of these fats. Sure, it's easy to eat bacon at every meal or put butter on top of everything, but that's not good nutrition. Maintaining a balance by eating a variety of fats is important to a nutritious keto diet. Plus, doing so adds tremendously to the "comfort" factor of this diet.

In addition to daily carb and calorie counts, the diet keeps track of the fat grams you eat each day. Each recipe provides fat grams, as do the daily menu plans.

FATS AND OILS TO AVOID

Although the Keto Comfort Food Diet is high in fat, this doesn't give you license to slather on every fat you meet. All fats are not created equal, even in keto nutrition. Steer clear of these unhealthy fats:

HYDROGENATED AND PARTIALLY HYDROGENATED OILS. Avoid any food or food product that contains "partially hydrogenated vegetable oil," a source of trans fats. Trans fats attach to a certain part of your cells that signals your DNA to oppose fat-burning, decelerate your metabolism, and make your body more resistant to insulin. Always check the ingredient list at the bottom of the label and avoid anything "hydrogenated." Fortunately, these nasty fats are being phased out of foods.

CERTAIN VEGETABLE OILS. These include corn oil, peanut oil, canola oil, soybean oil, and sunflower oil. These veggie oils are detrimental to your health—for a number of reasons. They're typically made from genetically modified seeds that are potential allergens. They easily go rancid (which carries health risks). They leave fatty deposits in your arteries that can lead to heart attacks. And they promote chronic inflammation in the body.

KETO COMFORT NUTS, SEEDS, AND BUTTERS

Nuts, seeds, and their associated flours and butters are another terrific source of healthy fats. These foods can sharpen your brain function, bolster your immune system, and help with digestion and blood-sugar control. They also have a moderate amount of protein and are generally low in carbs.

These foods are thus an important part of a healthful diet. Cooking with nuts adds a rich meatiness and a crunchy flavor to many dishes. Ethnic cuisines have long used nuts in dishes. Indians use cashews and almonds, while in Thailand people make extensive use of candlenuts and peanuts in their distinctive and aromatic style of cooking. And pesto with pine nuts is a traditional Mediterranean sauce.

Consisting of good monounsaturated fats, nuts have been found in numerous large studies to lower heart disease risk, improve blood-sugar and insulin control, and whittle your waist (as long as you don't binge on them!). Could nuts be better than a bottle of pills? Quite possibly!

And the benefits go beyond monounsaturated fat. Nuts are also high in fiber and protein.

As is often the case with nutrition recommendations, consume nuts in moderation because they are super high in calories. Though low in carbs, those carbs can add up if nuts are eaten in excess.

Also keto-friendly are butters made from nuts—not just peanut butter but also almond, cashew, Brazil, and macadamia nut butters—all without added sugar. These are delicious when incorporated into keto baked goods or keto candies.

I recommend that you eat 1 serving of nuts, seeds, nut flour, or nut butter daily. Here's a look at the daily serving sizes of these foods along with carb counts.

NUTS AND NUT BUTTERS	SERVING SIZE	CARBOHYDRATES (GRAMS)
Almonds	25 nuts	5.6
Almond butter	1 tablespoon	3.4
Almond flour or meal	2 tablespoons	3
Brazil nuts	6 nuts	3.5
Cashews	18 nuts	8.6
Cashew butter	1 tablespoon	4.4
Coconut meat	1 piece (2 x 2 x ½-inch)	7
Coconut, shredded (unsweetened)	¼ cup	5
Coconut flour	2 tablespoons	9
Hazelnuts	14 nuts	14
Macadamia nuts	12 nuts	4
Peanuts	2 tablespoons	3
Peanut butter	1 tablespoon	3
Pecans	2 tablespoons	2
Pine nuts	¼ cup	4.5
Pistachios	25 nuts	4
Walnuts	14 halves	4

I love experimenting with whole seeds to create keto comfort recipes. Not only can they be easily sprinkled atop many of your keto meals for a sneaky protein boost, they can also be cooked or baked into recipes.

You'll notice that I favor several different types of seeds. One is chia seeds. These tiny nutrition dynamos are so fiber rich that they can help with fullness and lead to weight loss. I use them raw, sprinkled on salads, in smoothies, or to make puddings. They also can be added to soups or baked in cookies.

I also love hemp seeds, which are super low in carbs compared with other seeds. When most people think of hemp, they associate it with getting high or a Cheech and Chong movie. But the only buzz you'll get from nutritional hemp is confidence that you're nurturing your body with its wealth of healthful contents: good fats, anti-inflammatory compounds, fiber, and amino acids.

With their rich nutty flavor, flaxseeds can improve the taste of keto breads, cookies, muffins, and grain-free cereals. Flaxseeds contain ALA, an omega fatty acid that cannot be produced by the body. They are also loaded with lignans, a type of phytochemical known to have cancer-protective power. Flaxseeds are packed with fiber, which fights constipation and helps normalize cholesterol. This type of fiber may also help with blood-sugar management, important for those with diabetes.

Then there are pumpkin seeds, also known as pepitas. They are a nutritional treasure trove of vitamins, minerals, and fiber essential for health and well-being. They are also involved in hormone balancing. I like to toss them into smoothies, salads, and even my Mushroom-Cauliflower Risotto (page 239).

I'd be remiss if I didn't mention sesame seeds, which have been popular in cooking for a very long time. Although sesame seeds are primarily grown in Southeast Asia and Africa, they are used practically everywhere throughout the world, from Sweden to Argentina.

My favorite form of sesame seeds comes as tahini, a paste of ground, hulled sesame seeds. You probably know it as an ingredient in hummus, but it's also having its moment in the world of confections, cookies, condiments, smoothies, salad dressings, and all sorts of dishes—even keto versions.

Back to hummus for a second: If you love hummus but know that you can't eat the traditional chickpea version on keto, don't worry. You can make hummus from mashed cauliflower and other nonstarchy vegetables. Simply add tahini and you're all set. See my hummus recipes on pages 181 and 182.

Here are the recommended serving sizes (1 serving daily) for seeds and seed butters along with carb counts.

SEEDS AND SEED BUTTERS	SERVING SIZE	CARBOHYDRATES (GRAMS)
Chia seeds	1 ounce	12.4
Flaxseeds, whole	2 tablespoons	7
Flaxseeds, ground	2 tablespoons	4
Hemp seeds	1 tablespoon	1
Hemp seed butter	1 tablespoon	2
Pumpkin seeds, hulled	1 ounce (142 seeds)	5
Sesame seeds	1 tablespoon	2
Sunflower seeds	1 tablespoon	2
Sunflower seed butter	1 tablespoon	4
Tahini	1 tablespoon	3

KETO COMFORT MEAT, POULTRY, AND SEAFOOD

Protein is well known for its ability to help you feel full. After eating a meal with protein, you'll feel satisfied and you'll be less likely to raid the fridge for something fattening. Protein increases your body's sensitivity to the hormone leptin, which tells your brain you're full and don't need any more food. And, of course, protein helps you retain lean, calorie-burning muscle as you lose weight.

I'm kind of harping on this but it's important: Many first-time keto dieters go whole hog (excuse the pun) on protein. But remember that a keto diet is not a high-protein diet; it's a moderate-protein diet. Too much protein is a major (and overlooked) no-no on the ketogenic diet. Your body can actually turn protein into glucose, so eating too much of the stuff can pull you out of ketosis and back into sugar-burning mode.

Very few proteins are off limits on the Keto Comfort Food Diet. Here is a list of allowable proteins.

Beef, including steaks, tenderloin, loin cuts, veal, roasts, and ground beef

Poultry (dark and white meats), including chicken, Cornish hens, quail, duck, turkey, ground poultry, and wild game

Pork, including pork loin, tenderloin, chops, ham, bacon (just make sure it contains no added sugar such as maple syrup), sausage, and ground pork

Fish of all types, especially mackerel, tuna, salmon, sardines, anchovies, sea bass, trout, halibut, cod, catfish, and redfish

Shellfish, including shrimp, oysters, clams, crab, mussels, and lobster

Organ meats, such as heart, liver, tongue, and kidney

Eggs

Lamb, including chops and roasts

These protein foods have zero or negligible carbs.

You should track your grams of protein daily; this amounts to 3 to 6 ounces of protein at each main meal. If you're a woman, your protein serving will be in the 3-ounce range; for a man, in the 6-ounce range. The meal plans ensure that you eat protein in the right ratios relative to the other macronutrients.

PROTEINS TO AVOID

To be successful on my plan, it's not only about eating the right amount of protein; it's also about eliminating the junk. Many meats are highly processed, such as cured meats, hot dogs, some luncheon meats, and certain types of jerky. Eating meats like these results in less intake of essential minerals. Consuming real chicken, fish, or meat, for example, typically supplies more than twice the potassium and magnesium found in processed luncheon meats containing the same amount of protein. Processed meats also contain additives, artificial ingredients, and unnecessary sugars—another reason to avoid them.

KETO COMFORT
NONSTARCHY VEGETABLES

While following the Keto Comfort Food Diet, eat plenty of nonstarchy vegetables. They are extremely important on this plan. The nutrients in fresh, organic vegetables help our bodies to not only survive but thrive. Don't worry, this doesn't mean that you have to eat the same old salad or steamed broccoli every day. There are lots of veggies you can eat, all prepared in so many delicious ways that you'll never get bored.

Vegetables are brimming with attributes. They pack a lot of fiber and water; both are "satiating." Satiating foods fill you to the point that you choose to stop eating. They work like a natural gastric bypass; you get full more quickly and automatically eat less. They are super low in carbs, making them perfect for triggering ketosis. Plus, they're loaded with vitamins, minerals, and phytochemicals.

I love to emphasize cabbage-family veggies such as broccoli, cabbage, cauliflower, and Brussels sprouts—otherwise known as the cruciferous vegetables. They take this unusual name from their "cross-shaped" flower petals. They are definitely fat-burning veggies—for several reasons.

First, they deliver glucosinolates, compounds involved in helping the liver detoxify drugs, pollutants, and other toxins. The liver is the main organ of metabolism. You need it running in peak form in order to burn fat. These veggies support liver function.

Second, all of these veggies are satiating because they're packed with fiber and water. They fill you up without filling you out. When these veggies are included in a meal or snack, you're less likely to eat higher-calorie, more fattening foods.

Third, cruciferous vegetables contain indole-3-carbinol (I3C), a natural compound that stops the growth and expansion of fat cells, according to a 2013 study reported in the *International Journal of Obesity*.

And finally, cruciferous vegetables contain a natural ingredient called 3,3′-Diindolylmethane (DIM) that destroys fat-forming foreign synthetic estrogens in the body. These estrogens come from various sources, including gasoline fumes, plastics, medicines, pesticides, and perfumes—any product that comes from petrochemical manufacturing. Foreign estrogens also come from our food supply. Hormones fed to cows and chickens to fatten them up are estrogen. It seems logical to suppose that eating hormone-dosed meat would have the same fattening effect on us.

Foreign estrogens thus accumulate in your body from constant exposure to environmental toxins and cause fat storage. They are the reason women are storing more belly fat today, and men have chronically lower testosterone levels.

Go for lots of green leafy vegetables, too. Think lettuce, spinach, kale, arugula, turnip greens, and mustard greens. They're full of fiber and antioxidants, and are very filling.

But they're full of something else: thylakoids, one of the components of chloroplasts, the parts of the plant cells used in photosynthesis. Photosynthesis is the process of converting sunlight into biochemical energy. Primarily found in the leaves of plants, thylakoids regulate appetite-regulating hormones, suppress food intake, normalize blood lipids, and decrease body weight in animals and humans.

In one study, a test group of 15 people who took supplemental thylakoids reported that it was easier to resist the temptation to eat between meals. Thylakoids slow down the digestion of fat, tricking stomachs into believing they have eaten enough. Foods containing thylakoids also prevent your body from releasing very high amounts of insulin (a fat-forming hormone), according to a study in the *Scandinavian Journal of Gastroenterology*. This is an important finding, since chronically high levels of insulin lead to fat gain and health risks.

How do you know if a veggie is high in thylakoids? If it's green, it's got 'em.

Make room for at least one, moderate-sized mixed salad several days during the week. And don't forget the celery and cucumbers!

Toss handfuls of spinach or kale into your smoothies, too. Anytime you can increase your intake of leafy greens, expect to see your scale gift you with ever-decreasing numbers.

Even though nonstarchy vegetables are low in carbs, you still have to watch your portions. If you eat too much of these, you may go over the carb limit. Example: 1 cup of kale contains around 7 grams of carbs, but if you ate a super big kale salad (with 3 or 4 cups of this veggie), the carbs in that salad will weigh in at well over 20 grams.

Eating a wide variety of vegetables guarantees that you're obtaining plenty of nutritional goodness and that you're not shortchanged of any one nutrient.

Enjoy the following veggies on my Keto Comfort Food Diet.

CARBOHYDRATES IN NONSTARCHY VEGETABLES

NONSTARCHY VEGETABLES	SERVING SIZE	CARBOHYDRATES (GRAMS)
Arugula	1 cup raw	1
Asparagus	½ cup cooked	3.5
Beet greens	½ cup cooked	4
Bell peppers	½ pepper	5
Bok choy	½ cup cooked	1.5
Broccoli	½ cup cooked 1 cup raw	4.5 6
Brussels sprouts	½ cup cooked	5.5
Butternut squash	½ cup cooked	10
Cabbage, all types	½ cup cooked 1 cup raw	3.5 4
Cauliflower	½ cup cooked 1 cup raw	2.5 6
Celery	3 stalks	4
Collard greens	½ cup cooked 2 large leaves	4 2
Cucumbers	1 cup sliced, raw, with peel	4
Eggplant	1 cup cooked cubes	8
Endive	1 cup chopped, raw	<1
Garlic	2 cloves	2
Green beans	½ cup cooked	5
Jalapeños	1 pepper	1
Kale	½ cup cooked 1 cup raw	3.5 7
Leeks	1 cup cooked	2
Lettuce, all types	1 cup raw	1.5
Mushrooms	½ cup cooked 1 cup sliced, raw	4 3
Mushrooms, portobello	1 large, grilled	5

NONSTARCHY VEGETABLES	SERVING SIZE	CARBOHYDRATES (GRAMS)
Mustard greens	½ cup cooked	3
Okra	½ cup cooked	4
Onion	½ cup sliced, raw	5.5
	¼ cup cooked	5
Radishes	6 radishes	1
Scallions/green onions	3 scallions	1
Shallots	3 tablespoons, chopped, raw	5
Spaghetti squash	½ cup cooked	5
Spinach	½ cup cooked	3.5
	1 cup raw	1
Sprouts	1 cup raw	1
Summer squash	1 cup cooked	4.5
Swiss chard	½ cup cooked	3.5
Tomatoes	1 tomato	5
Tomatoes, stewed	½ cup	3
Turnip greens	½ cup cooked	3
Yellow wax beans	½ cup cooked	2.5
Zucchini	½ cup cooked	4.5

VEGETABLES TO AVOID

Not all veggies are good for you on a keto diet. Focus on the nonstarchy vegetables listed above—and most other vegetables that grow above ground. Avoid high-carb vegetables such as potatoes, sweet potatoes, turnips, and beets. These are high-starch, high-carbohydrate vegetables that can boot you out of ketosis. You'll be able to enjoy these foods in maintenance, however.

KETO COMFORT FRUITS

While on my plan, you'll find that most fruits are on a "banned list." That's because many fruits contain excessive carbs and sugar, which can bring the fat-burning process to a frustrating halt.

One of the best fruits to include, however, are berries, mainly because they are low in carbs. Plus, they look gorgeous, taste delicious, and are definitely keto-friendly. Berries are naturally satiating because they're loaded with fiber. With a food I love, like fresh blueberries, for example, I've been known to eat past a feeling of satiety for the sake of sheer deliciousness.

Next, there's the thermogenic effect of berries. These tiny fruits contain the phenolic compound resveratrol (also in grapes and red wine), which increases heat in the body, burning calories in the process. Berries also contain carnitine, which assists muscle metabolism and is involved in burning fat. By incorporating more berries into your diet, you have a better chance of getting rid of stubborn body fat.

There are lots of other benefits to eating berries. They help in detoxifying the liver and lowering cholesterol and blood-sugar levels. They help cut the risk of heart attacks. And they enhance brain coordination and protect against age-related memory loss. Because berries are low in calories and carbohydrates and have a high fiber content, they are a popular food choice for a healthy diet.

Besides berries, there are other fruits you can enjoy on the plan.

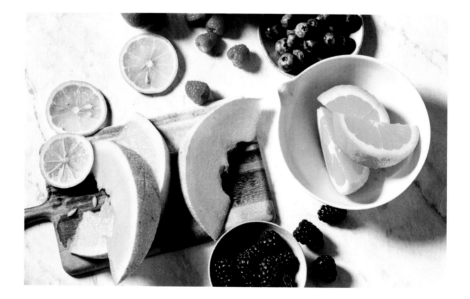

CARBOHYDRATES IN KETO-FRIENDLY FRUITS

KETO-FRIENDLY FRUITS	SERVING SIZE	CARBOHYDRATES (GRAMS)
Blackberries	½ cup	7
Blueberries	½ cup	10.5
Cantaloupe	¼ fruit	6
Cherries	½ cup	11
Cranberries	½ cup	6
Grapefruit	½ fruit	10
Lemon	1 fruit with peel	5
Lime	1 fruit with peel	7
Raspberries	½ cup	6.5
Watermelon	1 cup diced	11

FRUITS TO AVOID

Other fruits are off limits because they're high in carbs: apples, bananas, grapes, pine-apple, peaches, pears, and mangoes, to name just a few. Stick to the fruits listed above, but consider them a treat.

OTHER PLANT-BASED FOODS TO AVOID

To stay in ketosis, there are several otherwise healthy plant-based foods that you'll want to eliminate—until you get to your goal weight and can go on my maintenance plan.

Grains: All wheat (bread, pasta, cereal, bulgur, etc.), corn, oats, rice, buckwheat, millet, quinoa, barley, and so on

Vegetable-based pastas

Processed high-starch, high-sugar foods

Legumes and lentils

Sweets

KETO COMFORT DAIRY

Full-fat dairy foods are staples on ketogenic diets, so if you're a dairy lover you can enjoy many options. I love the fact that with the Keto Comfort Food Diet, I can welcome cheese back into my diet and not worry about what it does to my weight. There are far too many cheeses in the world to cover here (and definitely not enough time to enjoy them all!), but they all have their place on the plan.

There are fresh cheeses, for example. Ricotta is one of my favorites to use in cooking. There's just so much you can do with it: Use it as a base for dips, fill manicotti shells, layer it with eggplant "noodles," or make my Ricotta Cheesecake with Strawberry Sauce (page 283). Goat cheese is another preference, delicious when spiced or rolled in grape leaves.

I love to use many types of other cheeses in my recipes. Parmesan in chicken parm . . . blue cheese in salad dressings . . . mozzarella in all things Italian . . . cheddar shredded over lettuce tacos. There's no end to the uses and no cheese in which you can't indulge.

But please don't go overboard. If you consume too much dairy, you might find that you aren't burning fat fast enough. To lose weight you still need to watch your calorie intake somewhat. Because most dairy is packed with calories, it's very easy to consume so much that you go over the number of calories that your body needs to burn that day, which means that your body will convert the surplus calories to fat. So while you can eat cheese, you don't get to sit down and consume a whole block of cheddar.

A lot of people are already avoiding dairy because they're lactose intolerant or they want to avoid indirect exposure to the synthetic hormones and antibiotics injected into dairy cows to boost milk production. That's perfectly okay; you can be successful with keto if you exclude dairy. You can obtain your calcium from nondairy sources such as kale and collard greens, as well as from cruciferous veggies like Brussels sprouts and broccoli. What's more, you can also get calcium from sardines, shrimp, crab, and calcium-fortified nondairy milks.

If you still love dairy and want to include it, make sure to purchase only organic versions.

Enjoy these dairy foods in moderation.

CARBOHYDRATES IN KETO-FRIENDLY DAIRY FOODS

FULL-FAT DAIRY	SERVING SIZE	CARBOHYDRATES (GRAMS)
Asiago cheese	1 ounce (1-inch cube)	0
Blue cheese	1 ounce (1-inch cube)	<1
Brie	1 ounce (1-inch cube)	<1
Cheddar	1 ounce (1-inch cube)	<1
Coconut milk,* unsweetened	2 tablespoons	1
Colby cheese	1 ounce (1-inch cube)	0.4
Cottage cheese	½ cup	3
Cream cheese	2 tablespoons	1.2
Crème fraîche	2 tablespoons	0.5
Edam	1 ounce (1-inch cube)	0.4
Gouda	1 ounce (1-inch cube)	0.6
Kefir	½ cup	6
Monterey Jack	1 ounce (1-inch cube)	<1
Mozzarella, fresh	1-ounce ball	0
Mozzarella, shredded or grated	1 ounce	<1
Muenster	1 ounce (1-inch cube)	<1
Parmesan, shredded or grated	1 tablespoon	<1
Pecorino	1 ounce (1-inch cube)	0
Provolone	1 ounce (1-inch cube)	0.4
Ricotta cheese, whole-milk	½ cup	3
Swiss cheese	1 ounce (1-inch cube)	1
Whipping cream, heavy	1 tablespoon	0.4
Yogurt, Greek, plain	1 cup	4

* Coconut milk is not technically a dairy food; it's a nut milk.

DAIRY TO AVOID

A number of dairy foods contain sugar and starches and are not a good idea if you're trying to stay in ketosis. Avoid the following: low-fat, reduced-fat, and fat-free milk; half and half; evaporated and condensed milk.

WATER AND OTHER KETO COMFORT BEVERAGES

Now that I've covered foods you can chew, let's talk about keto-friendly beverages. The best is plain ol' water—and lots of it.

Drinking a lot of water wasn't hard for me on keto, since I'm in the habit of doing so. You need more water each day than any other nutrient. This is because water makes up about 60 percent of your body weight. Found in every cell, tissue, and organ in your body, water transports nutrients to cells, removes toxins from your body, lubricates your joints, and regulates your body temperature.

While following a keto diet, your body handles water differently, potentially causing dehydration. This tends to occur mostly during the fat adaptation stage as your body is converting from carbs for energy. As a result, your daily water requirements are higher than usual.

Here's what's going on: On a regular diet, your body likes to use carbs for fuel. Those carbs are converted to glucose for immediate use, and the remainder is converted to glycogen and stored in muscles and the liver. This stored glycogen is in a hydrated form; that is, there are 3 to 4 grams of water per 1 gram of glycogen. When carbohydrates are eliminated from the diet, or severely restricted, these glycogen stores are emptied quite rapidly, along with the accompanying water. This process often results in dehydration. Also, the keto diet eliminates many other sources of water, like fruits.

With this accelerated depletion of water, you must drink more liquids than usual. A good rule of thumb is to drink at least eight 8-ounce cups of water daily, or ten 8-ounce glasses daily if you work out intensely most days of the week.

If you don't stay hydrated, your body is going to store fat—which is the opposite of what you want. That's because adequate hydration also supports fat-burning. In research conducted at Humboldt University in Arcata, California, drinking a little over two 8-ounce glasses of water jacked up the metabolic rate by 30 percent in just 10 minutes.

Water is also satiating. Researchers at Virginia Tech found that people who drank water before meals lost more weight than those who did not. Often, thirst pangs are mistaken for hunger—so the next time you find yourself craving a snack in your midafternoon slump, drink a large glass of water first and see how you feel. The oxygen content in water (H_2O) also offers your brain and body a mini energy boost and aids in detoxification. Try to keep water always with you so you're not without it for too long.

Besides plain water, there are a lot of delightful drinks you can enjoy while following the Keto Comfort Food Diet.

Water with a few berries or cucumber slices to give it more flavor

Water with a squeeze or two of lemon or lime

Sparkling water or club soda, garnished with a lemon or lime wedge or a strawberry

Unsweetened plant-based milks like almond and coconut milk. (One cup of plant-based milk contains between 1 and 8 grams of carbs, so be sure to count those in your daily total.)

Coffee

Tea, including green tea and herbal teas

ALCOHOL AND KETO COMFORT

On most keto diets, alcohol isn't allowed, but because we're talking comfort here, you don't have to swear off alcohol. It does come with a few caveats, however.

Alcohol diminishes your inhibitions, causing you to overeat the wrong foods—which can put on pounds. Alcohol also turns off your liver's ability to burn fat. When alcohol enters the body, the liver drops its job of fat-burning and starts metabolizing the alcohol instead—like a worker who is pulled off an important job.

Alcohol can also be high in carbs, which will stop ketosis. You may also get tipsy more quickly while on a keto diet, and end up with a hangover that's worse than usual, because your body is running on fewer carbs.

If you like to imbibe occasionally, here are some alcoholic beverages that are the lowest in carbs.

LIQUORS (THESE HAVE 0 GRAMS OF CARBS)

Brandy	*Gin*	*Scotch*	*Vodka*
Cognac	*Rum*	*Tequila*	*Whiskey*

WINE (5-OUNCE SERVING)

Cabernet Sauvignon, 3.8 g *Pinot Grigio, 3.2 g*
Champagne, 1.5 g *Pinot Noir, 3.4 g*
Chardonnay, 3.7 g *Sauvignon Blanc, 2.7 g*
Merlot, 3.7 g

BEER (12-OUNCE SERVING)

Bud Select 55, 1.9 g *Rolling Rock Green Light, 2.4 g*
Michelob Ultra, 2.6 g

Be sure to check out my keto comfort food "kocktails" on pages 145 to 148.

ALCOHOL TO AVOID

Don't be tempted by the following drinks. They will send your blood sugar through the roof and stop ketosis.

Mojitos (except for mine on page 145), Cosmopolitans, rum and Cokes, Tom Collins, screwdrivers, gin and tonics, Long Island iced teas, and other mixed drinks; also avoid frozen drinks like piña coladas and margaritas (I have a keto version on page 147 that is allowed)

Regular beers and nonalcoholic beers, which can have as many as 18 grams of carbs per drink

Sweet wines like Riesling, Moscato, sweet sherry, and port, which average around 20 grams of carbs per glass

KEEP TRACK OF YOUR MACROS

If you plan some of your own meals or follow the meal plans here, it's important to calculate your calories, protein, fat, and carbohydrates in order to stay in ketosis. This involves a little simple math.

After planning your meals for the day, add up your daily calories, then tally up the daily grams of protein, fat, and carbs. Each gram of fat has 9 calories; each gram of protein or carbohydrate has 4 calories. So to figure out the percentages of macros in a day, here's the basic formula:

☐ Grams of protein for the day times 4 divided by your total daily calories equals your daily percentage of protein.

☐ Grams of fat for the day times 9 divided by your total daily calories equals your daily percentage of fat.

☐ Grams of carbohydrate for the day times 4 divided by your total daily calories equals your daily percentage of carbs.

Example: Your daily calories add up to 1,297. Your protein adds up to 74 grams, your fat to 103 grams, and your carbs to 22 grams. Here is the equation:

☐ Protein: $74 \times 4 = 296 \div 1{,}297 = 23\%$

☐ Fat: $103 \times 9 = 927 \div 1{,}297 = 71\%$

☐ Carbohydrate $22 \times 4 = 88 \div 1{,}297 = 7\%$

That's all there is to it.

I've made it easier with the meal plans in this book by doing the calculations for you. Be sure to keep weighing yourself periodically and testing your ketones to make sure that your percentages are on track and promoting ketosis.

I get it. I didn't particularly like math as a kid. In fact, to say I didn't like it would be like saying that being hit by a semitruck is an inconvenience. I couldn't stand it.

Fast-forward: I like math now. Being a chef, I had to juggle measurements of ingredients to create perfect dishes of delicious food. As a nutrition and diet author, I had to learn about calories and grams, and how they affect the body. I realized that being a good mathematical thinker is an important part of the food and nutrition territory.

Even so, for math haters who want to do some of their own meal planning, I've got an alternative. Just count one macro: carbohydrates. The rule of thumb is to stick to 30 grams of carbs or less.

If you're not losing weight or staying in ketosis at that range, you might be eating too much protein. Simply cut back a bit. Make sure you're eating at least 2 to 3 tablespoons of fat a day.

Try this keto hack and your body should stay in fat-burning mode in the absence of carbs.

CALORIES AND KETO

Do calories matter on the Keto Comfort Food Diet?

Yes, you need to curb calories on this plan in order to lose weight, although watching your macro percentages is the most important strategy. When people share their macros with me, the percentages are usually off. They're eating too much protein, for example, and that slows their progress. Carbs need to be low (around 30 grams or less), protein should be moderate, and fat should be higher than carbs or protein. When you cut carbs and keep protein at moderate levels, this automatically pushes calories lower.

Big red flag: I will say, however, if you totally gorge on fat—like eating a jar of peanut butter or a bag of pork rinds in one sitting—you will gain weight or halt your weight loss altogether. It's just common sense to not overindulge in any single food or food group. You can't eat as many calories as you want and lose weight on this plan or any ketogenic diet. If you are overeating, you will put on weight. It's as simple as that.

Here's the math of weight loss: 1 pound of fat = 3,500 calories. So, if you can engineer a deficit of 500 calories a day, you should theoretically lose 1 pound a week. The easiest way to reduce your normal calories by 500 per day is through diet and exercise. You can cut 250 calories from your diet and burn the remainder with extra exercise, for instance. Or, on more energetic days, you could exercise off 350 calories and eat 150 calories less. Weight loss just won't happen without calorie *and* macro control.

Tier 2 (the 21-day accelerated diet) is carefully calibrated to provide between 800 and 1,185 calories a day for rapid weight loss. Despite the lower calories, you won't feel hungry. That's because the macro percentages satiate you, meaning you won't get hungry or overeat. The fat and protein in the diet act like natural appetite suppressants.

So, when you're eating keto, you'll notice a natural decrease in your appetite, which is always helpful when you're trying to lose weight. You'll naturally end up eating less because you'll feel more satisfied with less food, and you'll no longer crave sugar.

Tier 3 (the basic 21-day diet) has a calorie range between 1,000 and 1,675 a day (depending on whether you eat keto desserts on any particular day). You'll still burn fat efficiently because you're staying in ketosis by keeping carbs low and dietary fat high.

GOING KETO IF YOU'RE A VEGAN
OR A VEGETARIAN

I'm often asked if it's possible to eat ketogenically while adhering to a vegan or vegetarian diet. For perspective, vegans don't eat meat, dairy, eggs, or anything that uses or contains animal products. Technically, a vegetarian is a person who doesn't eat meat but may eat dairy products such as cheese, milk, and eggs. A subgroup are lacto-vegetarians who eat dairy products such as milk, cheese, yogurt, butter, ghee, cream, and kefir, but exclude eggs. Ovo-vegetarians allow eggs but avoid dairy products—that's as animal as they get.

Although challenging, it's not impossible to go keto as a vegan or any type of vegetarian. There are basic eating habits to emphasize. Fats are a must. Choose vegetable-based fats and oil only, including olive oil, coconut oil, avocados, coconut cream, nuts, seeds, nut butters, and seed butters.

Protein is key, too. There are lots of plant-based options to choose from: nut milks (such as coconut milk and almond milk), seed milks (like hemp seed milk), vegan cheeses, cashew cheese, tofu, tempeh, coconut-based yogurt, vegan protein powder, and veggie burgers. I don't like to use fake meats in my recipes; I'd rather stick to natural plant-based proteins and a variety of fresh, organic, and seasonal ingredients. One more caveat: Even though tofu and other soy-derived foods are options, they contain plant estrogens that may interfere with fat loss. So these are foods you may want to avoid.

As with a regular keto diet, you'll have to remove all starchy carbs, including a lot of plant-based staples like beans, legumes, grains, and high-sugar fruits. Populate your diet with nonstarchy veggies: asparagus, lettuce, spinach, kale, greens of all varieties, cucumbers, cabbage, Brussels sprouts, broccoli, cauliflower, and the other vegetables I touched on earlier. On occasion, include berries as your primary fruit.

Stick to these guidelines and you can go keto as a vegan or a vegetarian.

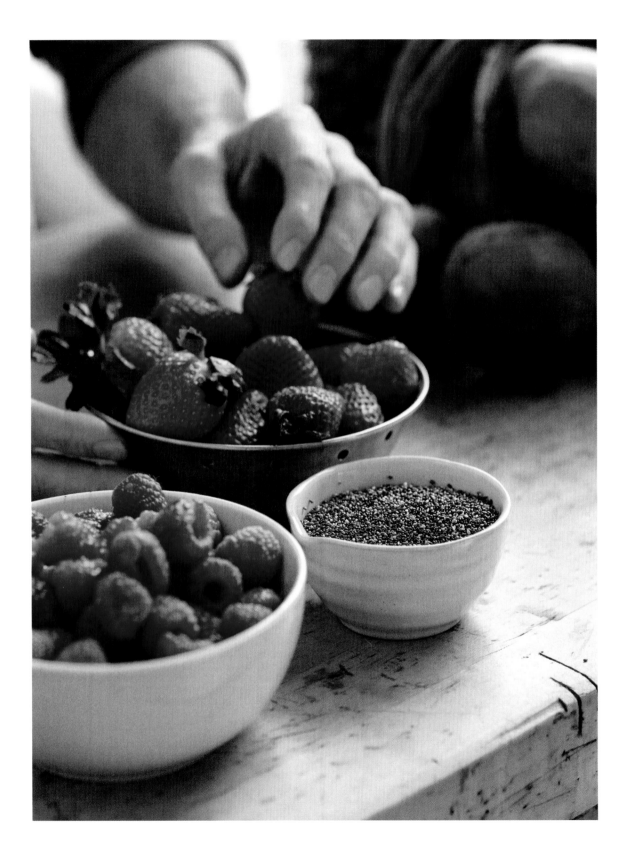

BEFORE YOU START . . .

To ensure your keto success, it's important to honestly assess where you are today. Once you know your true starting point, you'll be able to better form a clear vision of where you want to be. There are thus a couple of tasks I'd like you to do prior to starting this diet.

The first is to take "Before" pictures. One of the best ways to stay motivated is to be able to see tangible results—results that can't be disputed. So take several pictures of yourself first, and do it from different angles—front, side, and back. When you take the pictures, capture as much of your body as possible. Wear a bathing suit, ideally, and take the pictures against a plain background or white wall. If you don't want anyone to see you in a bathing suit, set your camera on a selfie stand, or pose in front of a full-length mirror, and snap away. Or have a family member or trusted friend take the photos.

Next, step on the scale and obtain your starting weight. Weigh yourself every few days at the same time each day to see how fast you're losing. Record those weights.

Remember that keto dieting burns pure fat. This means that you'll find yourself quickly losing inches. If your clothes are looser or fit better, that means inches are vanishing from your body, thanks to keto.

I recommend tracking the loss of those inches. At the very least, use a cloth tape measure to take the circumferences of your waist, hips, and thighs. To determine your waistline measurement, women should measure 1 inch above the navel and men should measure 1 inch below the navel. The tape measure should be snug, but should not compress the skin. Measure your thighs and hips at their widest part.

Let me add here that your waist measurement is a better tool than the number on your scale for monitoring health, says the National Heart, Lung, and Blood Institute. If you're a woman, shoot for a waist circumference of less than 36 inches; for men, it's less than 40 inches. The smaller your waist, the lower your risk for heart disease and type 2 diabetes.

Optional measurements include your chest, biceps, and calves. When measuring these body parts, measure at the widest parts.

Record these numbers in a journal or notebook.

Super important: Record your ketone bodies test results, too. Check your ketone levels in your urine, using test strips, in the morning and in the late afternoon.

When you take this time to honestly evaluate yourself, you've put yourself on the path to fat-burning.

PART TWO

KETO ON AND GET TRIM

TIER 1: THE 3-DAY KETO CLEANSE

The Keto Comfort Food Diet begins with my 3-Day Keto Cleanse designed to purify your body of all the processed carbs and sugar you may have been consuming and that have been causing you trouble. Carbs are sneaky. In excess, they tend to get converted to fat—which is why a rapid and strict carb cleanse is a good thing. It helps flush out bad stuff, expedite ketosis, and transition you to the full Keto Comfort Food Diet.

You will begin training your body for fat adaption, in which you depend on fat rather than carbs for energy. Relying on fat for fuel makes you feel more energetic. This is because carbohydrates, despite producing energy, trigger swings in blood sugar that result in drowsiness. Fat does not do this.

As you achieve fat adaption, you liberate yourself from carbohydrate dependence and train your body to burn fat.

The cleanse detoxes you of other bad stuff (besides processed carbs and sugar): bleached white flour, gluten, hydrogenated fats, genetically modified foods, and chemicals in our foods that can disrupt metabolism, make the liver less efficient, and pack on body fat.

This plan scrubs this stuff from your body and gently supports your body's own detoxification processes. It's also an excellent, useful way to launch the Keto Comfort Food Diet and ultimately build better long-term eating habits.

In the 3 days that you stay on the cleanse, don't be surprised if you drop 3 or more pounds. Read that again: 3 or more pounds in 3 days. Nice, isn't it? Yes, part of this will be excess water weight; the rest will be fat that needs to go.

I tested the cleanse on a group of dieters, and the results were phenomenal. Women lost an average of 4 pounds, and men lost even more. One man lost 8 pounds in 3 days! I instructed everyone to test their ketones once or twice daily. On average, by the third day, they had achieved ketosis. The cleanse was a hit, too. One dieter told me, "It was exactly what I needed to change the direction of the scale!"

Also important, the cleanse will leave you with a sense of confidence because you drop a lot of pounds right away. After finishing it, you will know that you can complete the 21-day diet and go on to reach your ideal weight.

All of this sounds great, doesn't it? Yes! Let's get started.

PREP FOR THE CLEANSE

Before you start, it's a good idea to "cleanse" your fridge and pantry. Toss out anything that might derail the Keto Cleanse, mainly processed carbs, sugar, and sweets. Tell your family and friends that you'll be cleansing and not available to go out for meals. It's only 3 days. You can do it.

The day before you begin, weigh yourself and record your weight. Don't weigh yourself again until the day after you finish the cleanse. Weight fluctuates like the stock market; stepping on the scale all the time and seeing fluctuations might frustrate you and distract you from the plan.

WHAT TO PURCHASE

Try to buy organic, fresh, seasonal vegetables whenever possible. You don't want to cleanse your body and then load it up with pesticides from conventionally grown produce. Switching to organic can have a quick and measurable impact on your health: Researchers at UC Berkeley found in 2019 that an organic diet can dramatically decrease the presence of many different pesticides in the urine of adults and children. Going organic applies to the 21-day plans, too.

Here is a sample shopping list for the cleanse. It is based on shopping for one person. Naturally, if others in your family are cleansing with you, you'll have to increase the amount of food you purchase. You may not need to purchase all of these items; it depends on what you decide to eat for dinner.

PROTEIN

Bacon, 6 slices

Beef marrow bones, 2½ pounds

Blue cheese crumbles

Chicken tenders

Eggs, ½ dozen

Parmigiano-Reggiano cheese

Tuna

VEGETABLES AND HERBS

1 yellow onion

2 carrots

Celery, 1 bunch

Garlic, 1 bulb

Parsley, 1 bunch

Thyme, 1 bunch

FATS

Unsalted grass-fed butter

Grass-fed ghee

MCT oil

OTHER

Apple cider vinegar

Coffee, herbal tea, or matcha tea

Granulated erythritol (optional)

Lemons

Spices and salad dressing ingredients
(see recipes for required items)

CLEANSE GUIDELINES

1. Pick 3 consecutive days when you can stick to the cleanse.

2. Make a batch of Keto Beef Bone Broth (page 241) ahead of time, since you'll be eating it for the 3 days of the cleanse. This is a high-electrolyte soup that helps prevent keto flu. Plus, it is extremely filling. You'll eat it at lunch, and you can have it as a snack if you feel hungry.

3. Follow the suggested meal plan that follows (pages 91 to 92), or feel free to improvise by choosing the salad you like best for dinner, or have a different salad each night.

4. You can have the salad at lunch and the broth at night (interchanging them), if you wish.

5. Do not deviate from the food choices. Stick to the foods on the meal plan. No fruit or carbs of any type.

6. If you feel hungry, nibble on celery sticks only, or have a cup of the bone broth.

7. Don't worry about cravings. They will not last. By day 3, you'll be fine. You'll begin to experience the positive effects of the cleanse—your sugar and salt cravings will subside, your taste buds will change, and you won't desire stuff you used to want.

8. Don't eat past 8 p.m. Food eaten after this time tends to take longer to digest because the body's metabolism slows down toward bedtime. Keep your system clear and working at its peak by avoiding late meals.

9. Drink eight to ten 8-ounce glasses of pure water throughout the day. Feel free to squeeze some fresh lemon juice into your water. Cups of green tea count and are encouraged. No alcohol or juices.

10. Weigh yourself before starting and after the final day.

11. Purchase keto test strips at the pharmacy. Test your urine twice through the day, upon arising and in the afternoon. You should see that you get into ketosis by the third day.

12. Do gentle exercise if you want to stay active during the cleanse. Walk, do some yoga, or engage in some light exercise. Movement stimulates the release of mood-lifting chemicals such as serotonin, endorphins, and dopamine, plus reins in your appetite and helps you stay energized. And if you sweat a little, that's good, too, since perspiration is an effective natural detoxifier that releases toxins through the skin.

13. If you feel tired, sleep. When you rest, your body has a chance to replenish and repair cells.

14. Don't stay on the cleanse longer than 3 days. However, you can use it again later—while on the diet or the maintenance plan—if you've gained weight and want to get back into ketosis quickly.

THE CLEANSE

Each day for 3 days, eat the following:

MEAL #1

Keto Breakfast Coffee (page 135)

Alternatives: Not a coffee drinker? Make the recipe with green tea or matcha. Both have a proven fat-burning record because they're thermogenic, meaning they rev up the body's calorie burn. Or choose coffee substitutes. Some good ones are Pero, Roma, Cafix, or Teeccino. Another option is to try maca tea, the legendary Peruvian super-food and energy and endurance booster.

MEAL #2

1 large bowl of Keto Beef Bone Broth (page 241)

Bone broth is a new superfood and used often in ketogenic diets. One of its benefits is that it supplies collagen. This is a protein found in our hair, bones, teeth, tendons, and cartilage that serves as connective tissue for the body cells. It supports healthier hair, skin, and nails, as well as a very important concern, a healthy gut. Bone broth may also protect the joints, help fight osteoarthritis, help reduce inflammation, aid sleep, and support weight loss.

Another nutrient in bone broth is calcium, an electrolyte that not only builds bone but also plays a big role in keeping the heart and muscles functioning properly. Bones used in bone broth also contain other minerals like magnesium (another electrolyte) and iron.

In general, studies show that a bowl of soup keeps you feeling full for longer, and good soups will speed your body's natural cleansing and detoxing system, helping your organs rid your body of the internal and environmental toxins that cause you to gain weight.

Bone broth is made by first roasting the bones from beef, pork, poultry (chicken or turkey), or fish, then boiling them for several hours until they break down and release protein and minerals. I add a bunch of veggies to mine for extra nutrition and flavor.

A keto comfort food salad—choose from the following:

☐ Basic quick keto salad (if you don't have time to make a salad recipe): Fresh greens, lettuce, salad veggies (raw broccoli, cauliflower, onions, grape tomatoes, bell peppers). Top with protein such as tuna, grilled chicken, or salmon. Drizzle with 2 tablespoons of MCT oil and apple cider vinegar.

☐ Tuna Salad over Bibb (page 204)

☐ Buffalo Chicken Salad (page 258)

☐ Kale and Spinach Caesar Salad (page 253)

☐ Classic Cobb Salad (page 254)

Veggies are particularly effective for cleansing purposes when consumed raw—that way, all of their natural fiber and nutrients are intact. Salads like these are also an especially enjoyable way to get your daily dose of vitamins. You might be skeptical that your appetite will be satisfied by a salad, but trust me, it will. To create a salad that will fill you up and burn fat, it's important to add some protein to your salad bowl—I've given you recipes that include protein.

After the 3-day cleanse is over—and you've completed it successfully—check in with yourself: How do you feel, mentally and physically? Did you notice that your stomach felt better after avoiding certain foods—or looked flatter? Do you feel lighter? How did your energy level fare? Did your skin clear up?

Doing the cleanse is an opportunity for real, live biofeedback: It gives you a chance to connect with your body and see how it's really feeling. Many people note that they have improved mental clarity, more energy, and better digestion after the cleanse.

And of course, now that you're done, it's time to get on the scale. Depending on your starting weight, you may find that you've lost up to 4 pounds (or more)—what a great way to kick off the next tiers of the Keto Comfort Food Diet.

Let's go!

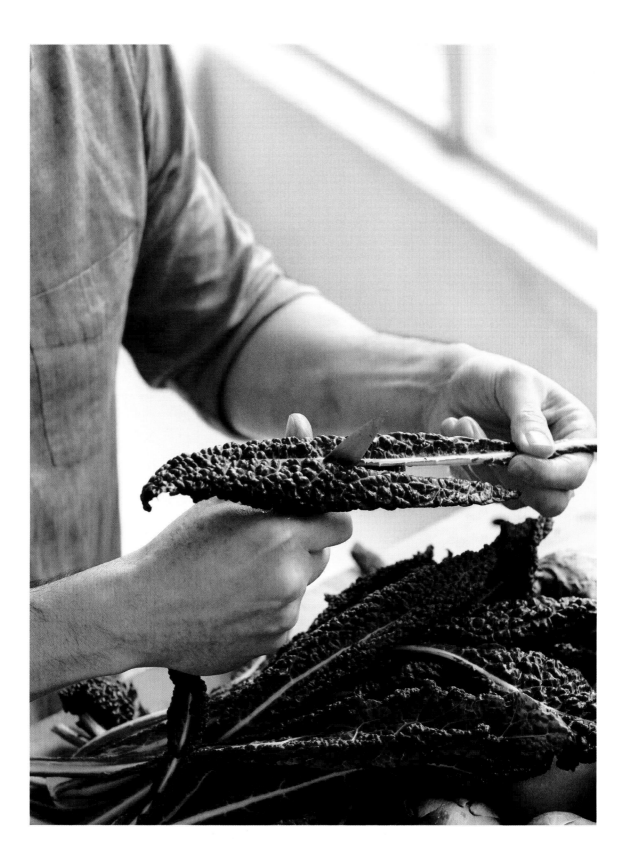

TIER 2: THE ACCELERATED 21-DAY KETO COMFORT FOOD DIET

Here's where you continue to burn fat at an impressive rate with the Accelerated Keto Comfort Food Diet and its meal plans. I give you 21 days of suggested daily menus, based on the recipes in Part 3.

This menu plan can be super helpful if you're just starting out and unsure about what you should be eating, or how much. The recipes make enough to allow leftovers, and I've incorporated those into the plan. If you don't prepare all the recipes, or desire something else, I provide suggestions for keto meals that can be substituted.

To begin, let me explain the accelerated plan in full.

INCORPORATE
INTERMITTENT FASTING

The accelerated tier emphasizes "intermittent fasting"—or taking periodic breaks from eating. This is a technique that puts your body into ketosis more quickly and naturally limits the amount of food you eat while on the plan. Here's how it works:

Go 16 hours without eating. The easiest way to do this is to fast overnight. If you finished your dinner at 8 p.m., for example, then your next meal of the day—lunch—would be at 12 p.m.

When you get up in the morning, have some lemon water (juice of a lemon squeezed into a cup of hot water), a cup of green tea, or a cup of black coffee. Then have your first meal at lunchtime. Another eating/fasting window can be early in the day—breakfast and lunch but no dinner.

Okay, I know what you're thinking! Isn't is totally wrong and unhealthy to skip breakfast? Isn't it the most important meal of the day? Won't skipping it make me hungrier later in the day?

No, no, and no.

Skipping breakfast, contrary to what you've been told, is perfectly okay. Various recent studies have found that going without breakfast does not hurt your metabolism, slow down fat-burning, or increase your appetite later in the day. In fact, skipping breakfast supports ketosis—the very fat-burning state you want to sustain.

Researchers Tanya and Eugene Zilberter reported in *Frontiers in Public Health* in 2014: "The supposed disadvantages of skipping [breakfast] have not been supported by recent controlled studies. . . . Perhaps it does not matter which of the daily meals—the first or the last—is omitted as long as at least once in a while, an inter-meal interval is long enough to allow the state of ketosis to initiate lipolysis [fat-burning] and lower calorie intake, thus decreasing the risk of obesity and its comorbidities [diseases related to obesity such as diabetes]." So, basically, intermittent fasting on occasion is a terrific way to initiate ketosis quickly and keep your body from gaining or regaining weight.

There are many scientifically recognized benefits of intermittent fasting: fat-burning, regulation of hunger hormones, reduced insulin resistance, faster metabolism, and less whole-body inflammation, among others. It is an excellent tool for achieving a lean, healthy body.

On Tier 2, there are no desserts, and the daily calorie counts are lower than on Tier 3.

Here is the Accelerated 21-day Keto Comfort Food Diet plan, along with recipes, calorie counts, and macro percentages. The shopping list for Tier 2 can be found in Appendix A.

WEEK 1

	CALORIES	PROTEIN (G)	FAT (G)	CARBS (G)	% PROTEIN	% FAT	% CARBS
DAY 1							
Black coffee, green tea, or lemon water	-	-	-	-	-	-	-
LUNCH: Asian-Marinated Flank Steak Stir-Fry (page 194)	295	38	10	11	53%	32%	15%
DINNER: Nut-Crusted Fish (page 235) with The Creamiest Coleslaw with Dill (page 257)	344 / 246	38 / 2	20 / 22	3 / 10	44% / 3%	52% / 81%	4% / 16%
SNACK: Chocolate Peanut Butter Fat Bombs (page 185)	122	3	12	3	9%	82%	9%
DAY 1 TOTAL	**1,007**	**81**	**64**	**27**	**32%**	**57%**	**11%**
DAY 2							
Black coffee, green tea, or lemon water	-	-	-	-	-	-	-
LUNCH: Leftover Asian-Marinated Flank Steak Stir-Fry (page 194)	295	38	10	11	53%	32%	15%
DINNER: Chicken Parmesan (page 225)	400	48	18	9	48%	41%	11%
SNACK: Chocolate Peanut Butter Fat Bombs (page 185)	122	3	12	3	9%	82%	9%
DAY 2 TOTAL	**817**	**89**	**40**	**23**	**44%**	**45%**	**11%**
DAY 3							
Black coffee, green tea, or lemon water	-	-	-	-	-	-	-
LUNCH: Classic Cobb Salad (page 254)	384	11	35	7	11%	82%	7%
DINNER: The Ultimate Meatloaf (page 236)	361	22	29	3	25%	72%	3%
SNACK: Cauliflower Hummus (page 182)	255	5	21	12	7%	75%	18%
DAY 3 TOTAL	**1,000**	**38**	**85**	**22**	**15%**	**77%**	**8%**

	CALORIES	PROTEIN (G)	FAT (G)	CARBS (G)	% PROTEIN	% FAT	% CARBS
DAY 4							
Black coffee, green tea, or lemon water	-	-	-	-	-	-	-
LUNCH: Leftover The Ultimate Meatloaf (page 236)	361	22	29	3	25%	72%	3%
DINNER: Shrimp and Cheesy Cauliflower Grits (page 226)	316	34	17	6	43%	49%	8%
SNACK: Cauliflower Hummus (page 182)	255	5	21	12	7%	75%	18%
DAY 4 TOTAL	**932**	**61**	**75**	**21**	**21%**	**65%**	**14%**
DAY 5							
Black coffee, green tea, or lemon water	-	-	-	-	-	-	-
LUNCH: Tuna Salad over Bibb (page 204)	393	37	23	4	38%	53%	9%
DINNER: Grilled sirloin steak and Cauliflower Mashed Potatoes (page 262)	259 / 217	43 / 4	8 / 21	0 / 3	72% / 7%	28% / 87%	0% / 6%
SNACK: Handful of almonds (25)	167	6	14	5	14%	75%	11%
DAY 5 TOTAL	**1,036**	**90**	**66**	**12**	**36%**	**58%**	**6%**
DAY 6							
Black coffee, green tea, or lemon water	-	-	-	-	-	-	-
LUNCH: Texas-Style Chili (page 249)	366	16	25	20	17%	61%	22%
DINNER: Hot Crispy Keto Fried Chicken (page 221) and Mustard Greens with Bacon, Garlic, and Ginger (page 265)	360 / 70	22 / 6	27 / 2	6 / 7	25% / 34%	68% / 26%	7% / 40%
SNACK: Handful of almonds (25)	167	6	14	5	14%	75%	11%
DAY 6 TOTAL	**963**	**50**	**68**	**38**	**20%**	**64%**	**16%**
DAY 7							
Black coffee, green tea, or lemon water	-	-	-	-	-	-	-
LUNCH: Mediterranean Salmon Burger (page 202) and Parmesan Herbed Zucchini Fries (page 270)	371 / 156	34 / 10	23 / 10	7 / 6	36% / 26%	56% / 58%	8% / 16%
DINNER: Low-Carb Butternut Squash Soup (page 246)	281	3	21	20	4%	67%	29%
SNACK: Herbed Parmesan Crisps (page 189)	133	12	8	2	36%	60%	4%
DAY 7 TOTAL	**941**	**59**	**62**	**35**	**25%**	**59%**	**16%**

	CALORIES	PROTEIN (G)	FAT (G)	CARBS (G)	% PROTEIN	% FAT	% CARBS
DAY 8							
Black coffee, green tea, or lemon water	-	-	-	-	-	-	-
LUNCH: Buffalo Chicken Salad (page 258)	400	19	33	8	19%	73%	8%
DINNER: Meat Lovers' Cauliflower Pizza (page 219)	386	28	26	10	29%	61%	10%
SNACK: Herbed Parmesan Crisps (page 189)	133	12	8	2	36%	60%	4%
DAY 8 TOTAL	**919**	**59**	**67**	**20**	**26%**	**66%**	**8%**
DAY 9							
Black coffee, green tea, or lemon water	-	-	-	-	-	-	-
LUNCH: Cajun Fish "Tacos" (page 198)	316	27	20	7	34%	57%	9%
DINNER: Sloppy Joe Pot Pie (page 232)	385	15	31	12	16%	72%	12%
SNACK: Avocado Hummus (page 181)	191	4	15	10	8%	71%	21%
DAY 9 TOTAL	**892**	**46**	**66**	**29**	**20%**	**67%**	**13%**
DAY 10							
Black coffee, green tea, or lemon water	-	-	-	-	-	-	-
LUNCH: Pork Fried Rice (page 208)	360	19	24	16	22%	60%	18%
DINNER: Mushroom-Cauliflower Risotto with Pepitas (page 239)	309	15	21	15	20%	60%	20%
SNACK: 1 ounce cheddar cheese	120	6	10	0	16%	84%	0%
DAY 10 TOTAL	**789**	**40**	**55**	**31**	**20%**	**64%**	**16%**
DAY 11							
Black coffee, green tea, or lemon water	-	-	-	-	-	-	-
LUNCH: Leftover Mushroom-Cauliflower Risotto with Pepitas (page 239)	309	15	21	15	20%	60%	20%
DINNER: Mama's Keto Meatballs with Zucchini Noodles (page 215)	400	32	21	20	32%	48%	20%
SNACK: 2 hard-boiled eggs	155	13	11	1	18%	70%	12%
DAY 11 TOTAL	**864**	**60**	**53**	**36**	**28%**	**55%**	**17%**

	CALORIES	PROTEIN (G)	FAT(G)	CARBS (G)	% PROTEIN	% FAT	% CARBS
Black coffee, green tea, or lemon water	-	-	-	-	-	-	-
LUNCH: Keto Comfort Bacon Burger (page 201)	400	26	33	6	20%	74%	6%
DINNER: Chicken and Dumpling Soup (page 243)	362	20	26	12	22%	65%	13%
SNACK: 2 celery sticks with 1 tablespoon almond butter	111	3	9	6	10%	70%	20%
DAY 12 TOTAL	**873**	**49**	**68**	**24**	**20%**	**70%**	**10%**
Black coffee, green tea, or lemon water	-	-	-	-	-	-	-
LUNCH: Leftover Chicken and Dumpling Soup (page 243)	362	20	26	12	22%	65%	13%
DINNER: Grilled sirloin steak and Spicy Bacon Brussels Sprouts (page 269)	259 / 145	43 / 6	8 / 9	0 / 10	72% / 16%	28% / 56%	0% / 28%
SNACK: Coconut-Strawberry Smoothie (page 143)	327	6	28	10	9%	78%	13%
DAY 13 TOTAL	**1,093**	**75**	**71**	**32**	**28%**	**60%**	**12%**
Black coffee, green tea, or lemon water	-	-	-	-	-	-	-
LUNCH: Buffalo Chicken Salad (page 258)	400	19	33	8	19%	73%	8%
DINNER: Pan-fried pork sirloin chop (boneless) and Braised Baby Bok Choy (page 273)	274 / 239	44 / 2	10 / 23	0 / 6	67% / 3%	33% / 87%	0% / 10%
SNACK: Slice of Berry Bread with Chia Seeds (page 152)	199	6	17	9	11%	72%	17%
DAY 14 TOTAL	**1,112**	**71**	**83**	**23**	**25%**	**67%**	**8%**

DAY 12

DAY 13

DAY 14

	CALORIES	PROTEIN (G)	FAT (G)	CARBS (G)	% PROTEIN	% FAT	% CARBS
DAY 15							
Black coffee, green tea, or lemon water	-	-	-	-	-	-	-
LUNCH: Shrimp Pad Thai (page 197)	302	29	14	17	38%	41%	21%
DINNER: Baked chicken thigh and Creamed Spinach (page 278)	296 / 274	37 / 4	15 / 26	0 / 6	54% / 6%	46% / 85%	0% / 9%
SNACK: Slice of Berry Bread with Chia Seeds (page 152)	199	6	17	9	11%	72%	17%
DAY 15 TOTAL	**1,071**	**76**	**72**	**32**	**28%**	**60%**	**12%**
DAY 16							
Black coffee, green tea, or lemon water	-	-	-	-	-	-	-
LUNCH: Herb and Garlic Salmon over Arugula (page 211)	421	26	33	6	25%	70%	5%
DINNER: Mushroom-Cauliflower Risotto with Pepitas (page 239)	309	15	21	15	20%	60%	20%
SNACK: Jalapeño Poppers with Bacon (page 186)	193	7	17	3	15%	79%	6%
DAY 16 TOTAL	**923**	**48**	**71**	**24**	**21%**	**69%**	**10%**
DAY 17							
Black coffee, green tea, or lemon water	-	-	-	-	-	-	-
LUNCH: Chicken and Cauliflower Tikka Masala (page 212)	422	17	34	13	16%	72%	12%
DINNER: Broccoli-Cheddar Soup (page 245)	382	17	30	11	18%	71%	11%
SNACK: Jalapeño Poppers with Bacon (page 186)	193	7	17	3	15%	79%	6%
DAY 17 TOTAL	**997**	**41**	**81**	**27**	**16%**	**73%**	**11%**
DAY 18							
Black coffee, green tea, or lemon water	-	-	-	-	-	-	-
LUNCH: Steak Fajita Platter with Peppers and Avocado Mash (page 205)	395	26	27	16	25%	60%	15%
DINNER: Ground Pork Ramen (page 250)	297	11	23	12	15%	69%	16%
SNACK: Guacamole with Pepitas and Pomegranate (page 190)	195	12	14	8	23%	61%	16%
DAY 18 TOTAL	**887**	**49**	**64**	**36**	**22%**	**64%**	**14%**

	CALORIES	PROTEIN (G)	FAT(G)	CARBS (G)	% PROTEIN	% FAT	% CARBS
DAY 19							
Black coffee, green tea, or lemon water	-	-	-	-	-	-	-
LUNCH: Tuna Salad over Bibb (page 204)	393	37	23	4	38%	53%	9%
DINNER: Mama's Keto Meatballs with Zucchini Noodles (page 215)	400	32	21	20	32%	48%	20%
SNACK: Guacamole with Pepitas and Pomegranate (page 190)	195	12	14	8	23%	61%	16%
DAY 19 TOTAL	**988**	**81**	**58**	**32**	**33%**	**54%**	**13%**
DAY 20							
Black coffee, green tea, or lemon water	-	-	-	-	-	-	-
LUNCH: Mediterranean Salmon Burger (page 202) and Parmesan Herbed Zucchini Fries (page 270)	371 156	34 10	23 10	7 6	36% 26%	56% 58%	8% 16%
DINNER: The Ultimate Meatloaf (page 236)	361	22	29	3	25%	72%	3%
SNACK: Spinach and Artichoke Dip (page 192)	284	9	24	8	13%	76%	11%
DAY 20 TOTAL	**1,172**	**75**	**86**	**24**	**26%**	**66%**	**8%**
DAY 21							
Black coffee, green tea, or lemon water	-	-	-	-	-	-	-
LUNCH: Kale and Spinach Caesar Salad (page 253)	315	8	29	5	10%	84%	6%
DINNER: The Ultimate Meatloaf (page 236) and Keto Dinner Roll (page 162)	361 222	22 11	29 17	3 5	25% 21%	72% 69%	3% 10%
SNACK: Spinach and Artichoke Dip (page 192)	284	9	24	8	13%	76%	11%
DAY 21 TOTAL	**1,182**	**50**	**99**	**21**	**17%**	**75%**	**8%**

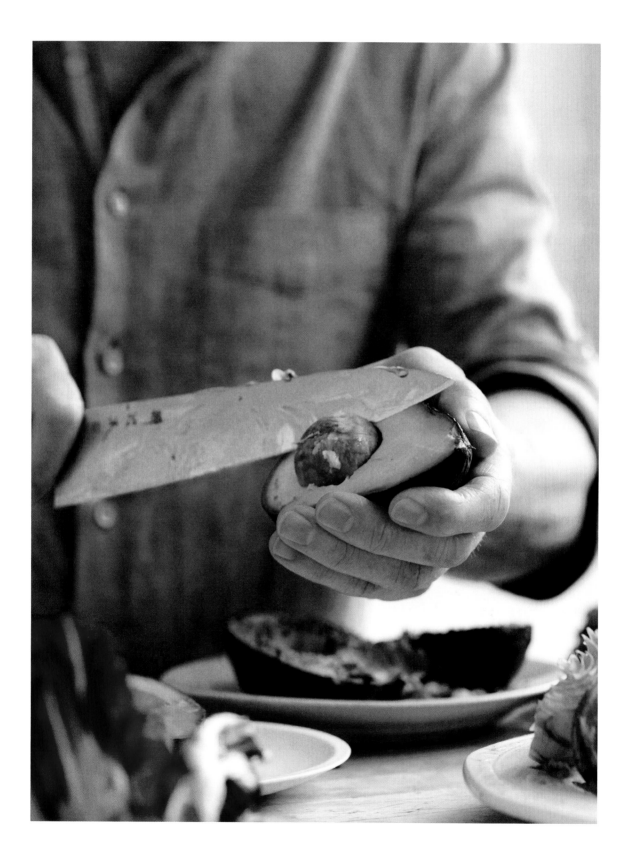

SUBSTITUTE YOUR OWN KETO COMFORT FOOD MEALS

One of the keys to success on the Keto Comfort Food Diet is to cook at home more often and eat out less. By cooking at home, you're in charge: of the ingredients, the calories, the sodium, the sugar, the fat, the portion size—everything that's important to your weight and health.

Okay—I've gone on the record to encourage home cooking, but I realize not everyone will buy in. So I want to help you put together some keto combinations that are quick and easy. First understand how to structure your meals.

BREAKFAST: You're not eating breakfast on Tier 2 so I'll cover that in the next chapter.

LUNCH: A protein + fat + nonstarchy vegetables (including a green leafy salad sprinkled with cheese or seeds and drizzled with oil). Sometimes, you can add in a grain-free "bread," "roll," "muffin," and so on (see pages 150 to 162).

DINNER: A protein + fat + nonstarchy vegetables (including a green leafy salad sprinkled with cheese or seeds and drizzled with oil).

KETO COMFORT FOOD SNACKS: You won't feel too hungry between meals—that's one of the big benefits of the Keto Comfort Food Diet. But if you do, snacking is allowed. Here are some fat-burning snacks.

Any recipe from the snack section (pages 180 to 192)

Cheese (1 ounce)

A handful of nuts or seeds

Cheese (1 ounce) with 3 to 4 olives

1 or 2 hard-boiled eggs

Any keto comfort food slushee or smoothie (pages 137 to 144)

Whole-milk plain Greek yogurt (1 cup) mixed with ½ cup berries

Cottage cheese (½ cup) mixed with ½ cup sliced strawberries

1 serving of any keto-friendly fruit (refer to the chart on page 71 for appropriate serving sizes)

Celery sticks with salsa (sugar-free) or guacamole

Celery sticks spread with nut butter

Raw veggies dipped in a keto comfort food hummus (pages 181 and 182)

Smaller portions of any leftover keto comfort food meal

PERSONALIZE YOUR DAILY MEALS

In addition to using the recipes suggested, you can also create "throw-together" meals and intersperse them in your plan with any of the recipes you like.

LUNCHES

THROW-TOGETHER

Turkey or beef burger topped with cheese, mushrooms, and avocado and wrapped in large lettuce leaves

Arugula salad with hard-boiled eggs, sliced turkey, avocado, and blue cheese dressing

Caesar salad topped with grilled salmon

Grilled chicken breast sautéed in olive oil with a sliced Roma (plum) tomato and 1 cup mixed greens

RECIPE-BASED

Any of the keto comfort food salads, soups, or stews (pages 240 to 259)

Any of the keto comfort food lunches (pages 193 to 213)

Any leftovers from the above options

DINNERS

THROW-TOGETHER

Grilled shrimp topped with a lemon butter sauce with a side of asparagus

Pork chop with mashed cauliflower and coleslaw

Grilled salmon or other fish served with a side of cauliflower and sautéed greens (or a keto comfort food side, pages 260 to 278)

Grilled steak with a side salad, drizzled with olive oil and vinegar, and any steamed low-carb veggie

RECIPE-BASED

Any keto comfort food dinner (pages 214 to 239) + a keto comfort food side (pages 260 to 278)

Any keto comfort food protein + a keto comfort food side

Any leftovers from the above options

To assist you in planning your meals on Tier 2, here is a daily worksheet that can be copied as needed and filled in.

BREAKFAST

_____

BLACK COFFEE, GREEN TEA, OR LEMON WATER
(SPECIFY WHICH YOU CHOOSE)

LUNCH

_____

KETO COMFORT FOOD LUNCH RECIPE

OR _____

    └ KETO COMFORT FOOD SALAD, SOUP, OR STEW RECIPE

OR _____

    ├ PROTEIN
    +
    ├ _____
    ├ NONSTARCHY VEGETABLES
    +
    └ FAT

DINNER

_____

KETO COMFORT FOOD DINNER RECIPE

OR _____

    ├ PROTEIN
    +
    ├ _____
    ├ NONSTARCHY VEGETABLES OR KETO
    │ COMFORT FOOD SIDE RECIPE
    +
    └ FAT

SNACK

_____

KETO COMFORT FOOD SNACK RECIPE

OR _____

    └ SNACK FROM THE APPROVED LIST

MY DAILY NUTRITION

_____

TOTAL CALORIES

_____

TOTAL GRAMS OF PROTEIN

_____

TOTAL GRAMS OF FAT

_____

TOTAL GRAMS OF CARBOHYDRATES

_____

DAILY PERCENTAGE OF PROTEIN

_____

DAILY PERCENTAGE OF FAT

_____

DAILY PERCENTAGE OF CARBOHYDRATES

Watch your portions when planning meals. The recipes are portion controlled for you, so you don't have to worry about measuring things out. The portion sizes of my recipes can also teach key lessons, like what a single portion of protein or veggies really should look like.

_____

_____

EXERCISE PORTION CONTROL

Portions are built into the recipes so you don't really have to measure. A good way to measure portions is by using your hand—no measuring cups, spoons, or scales needed. As reported in the *Journal of Nutritional Science,* a study from the University of Sydney in Australia tested this hand-measuring approach by having 67 people measure 42 foods and liquids with their finger widths and then using formulas to calculate the volume and weight of the items. This was found to be more precise than visualizing common household measures.

Here's how to use this "hands-on" method.

☐ Fist = 1 cup vegetables or fruit, such as chopped broccoli, whole small berries, or chopped fruit

☐ Thumb tip (from the second joint) = 1 teaspoon nut butter, butter, ghee, whipped cream, full-fat cream, olive oil, or coconut oil

☐ Whole thumb = 1 ounce cheese

☐ Flat palm = 3 to 4 ounces of fish, chicken, or meat. Larger palms represent 5 to 6 ounces (which is appropriate for a man's portion).

☐ Cupped hand = 1 to 2 ounces nuts

NON-HAND MEASUREMENTS OF SERVING SIZES

1 cup whole-milk plain yogurt

½ to 1 scoop protein powder

2 whole eggs

2 slices bacon

¼ to ½ avocado

1 tablespoon olives

1 average piece allowable fruit

TIER 2 GUIDELINES

I want you to burn fat rapidly, control your appetite, and achieve optimal health—and have a body-and-soul-satisfying experience in the process. Here are a few simple guidelines to make that happen on this tier.

1. Follow Tier 2 for 21 days. If you have more weight to lose, move on to Tier 3.

2. Make sure your daily carbohydrate counts stay around or under 30 grams. This helps ensure that your carb count stays in the ketosis-producing range.

3. Include protein, nonstarchy veggies, and fat at each main meal.

4. Follow the intermittent fasting strategy daily.

5. Avoid sugary and high-starch foods completely, as well as junk foods, processed foods, and low-fat foods.

6. Stay well hydrated.

7. Avoid alcohol, as well as any desserts, on this tier.

8. Review the shopping lists in Appendix A prior to going to the grocery store.

9. Choose organic for both produce and animal products if possible.

10. Study the recipes carefully prior to cooking. They are easy to prepare, even if you don't ordinarily do a lot of cooking.

11. Test yourself daily (in the morning and afternoon) to make sure you're staying in ketosis. Keep track of your weight loss every few days.

TIER 3: THE BASIC 21-DAY KETO COMFORT FOOD DIET

You've been following the plan for a little more than 21 days and I'm sure you're seeing much less of yourself, since junk carbs and sugary stuff are no longer packing on the pounds. I hope you love how trim you look, the compliments you're getting, and the ability to slide into your skinny jeans.

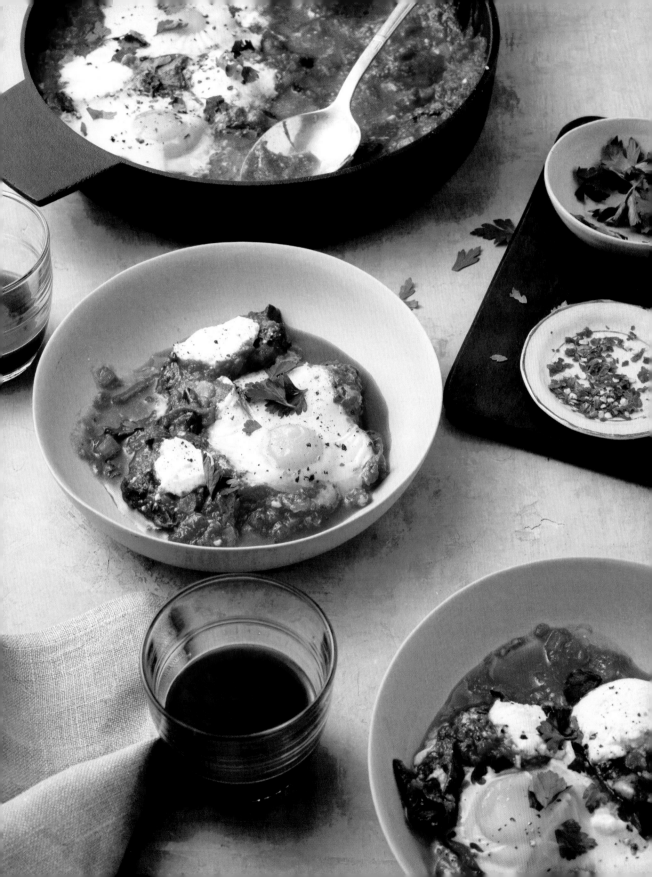

If you haven't reached your ideal weight yet, it's time to go on Tier 3. On this tier, you get to eat more calories (between 1,200 and 1,600), including breakfast and desserts (if you desire). Those three aspects of Tier 3 are what makes it different from Tier 2.

Here is the Basic 21-Day Keto Comfort Food Diet plan, along with recipes, calorie counts, and macro percentages. The shopping list for Tier 3 can be found in Appendix A.

TIER 3: THE BASIC 21-DAY KETO COMFORT FOOD DIET

WEEK 1

	CALORIES	PROTEIN (G)	FAT(G)	CARBS (G)	% PROTEIN	% FAT	% CARBS
DAY 1							
BREAKFAST: Peanut Butter Chocolate Slushee (page 137)	363	9	29	13	12%	73%	15%
LUNCH: Asian-Marinated Flank Steak Stir-Fry (page 194)	295	38	10	11	53%	32%	15%
DINNER: Nut-Crusted Fish (page 235)	344	38	20	3	44%	52%	4%
OPTIONAL DESSERT: Ricotta Cheesecake with Strawberry Sauce (page 283)	351	12	31	6	14%	79%	7%
SNACK: Chocolate Peanut Butter Fat Bombs (page 185)	122	3	12	3	9%	82%	9%
DAY 1 TOTAL (with dessert)	**1,475**	**100**	**102**	**36**	**27%**	**63%**	**10%**
DAY 1 TOTAL (without dessert)	**1,124**	**88**	**71**	**30**	**32%**	**57%**	**11%**
DAY 2							
BREAKFAST: Mixed-Berry Smoothie (page 139)	250	14	18	6	23%	66%	11%
LUNCH: Leftover Asian-Marinated Flank Steak Stir-Fry (page 194)	295	38	10	11	53%	32%	15%
DINNER: Chicken Parmesan (page 225)	400	48	18	9	48%	41%	11%
OPTIONAL DESSERT: Leftover Ricotta Cheesecake with Strawberry Sauce (page 283)	351	12	31	6	14%	79%	7%
SNACK: Chocolate Peanut Butter Fat Bombs (page 185)	122	3	12	3	9%	82%	9%
DAY 2 TOTAL (with dessert)	**1,418**	**115**	**89**	**35**	**33%**	**57%**	**10%**
DAY 2 TOTAL (without dessert)	**1,067**	**103**	**58**	**29**	**39%**	**50%**	**11%**

	CALORIES	PROTEIN (G)	FAT(G)	CARBS (G)	% PROTEIN	% FAT	% CARBS
DAY 3							
BREAKFAST: Spinach-Cantaloupe Slushee (page 138)	304	18	20	12	24%	60%	16%
LUNCH: Classic Cobb Salad (page 254)	384	11	35	7	11%	82%	7%
DINNER: The Ultimate Meatloaf (page 236)	361	22	29	3	25%	72%	3%
OPTIONAL DESSERT: Chocolate Avocado Mousse (page 280)	218	3	18	11	6%	74%	20%
SNACK: 1 ounce cheddar cheese	120	6	10	0	16%	84%	0%
DAY 3 TOTAL (with dessert)	**1,387**	**60**	**112**	**33**	**18%**	**73%**	**9%**
DAY 3 TOTAL (without dessert)	**1,169**	**57**	**94**	**22**	**20%**	**72%**	**8%**
DAY 4							
BREAKFAST: Chocolate-Glazed Doughnut (page 157)	241	4	21	9	7%	78%	15%
LUNCH: Leftover The Ultimate Meatloaf (page 236)	361	22	29	3	25%	72%	3%
DINNER: Shrimp and Cheesy Cauliflower Grits (page 226)	316	34	17	6	43%	49%	8%
OPTIONAL DESSERT: Ricotta Cheesecake with Strawberry Sauce (page 283)	351	12	31	6	14%	79%	7%
SNACK: Cauliflower Hummus (page 182)	255	5	21	12	7%	75%	18%
DAY 4 TOTAL (with dessert)	**1,524**	**77**	**119**	**36**	**20%**	**70%**	**10%**
DAY 4 TOTAL (without dessert)	**1,173**	**65**	**88**	**30**	**22%**	**68%**	**10%**
DAY 5							
BREAKFAST: Chocolate-Glazed Doughnut (page 157)	241	4	21	9	7	78%	15%
LUNCH: Tuna Salad over Bibb (page 204)	393	37	23	4	38%	53%	9%
DINNER: Grilled sirloin steak and Cauliflower Mashed Potatoes (page 262)	259 / 217	43 / 4	8 / 21	0 / 3	72% / 7%	28% / 87%	0% / 6%
OPTIONAL DESSERT: Cranberry Cherry Almond Crumble (page 295)	172	4	12	12	9%	63%	28%
SNACK: Handful of almonds (25)	167	6	14	5	14%	75%	11%
DAY 5 TOTAL (with dessert)	**1,449**	**98**	**99**	**33**	**28%**	**62%**	**10%**
DAY 5 TOTAL (without dessert)	**1,277**	**94**	**87**	**21**	**30%**	**62%**	**8%**

	CALORIES	PROTEIN (G)	FAT(G)	CARBS (G)	% PROTEIN	% FAT	% CARBS
BREAKFAST: Mixed-Berry Smoothie (page 139)	250	14	18	6	23%	66%	11%
LUNCH: Broccoli-Cheddar Soup (page 245)	382	17	30	11	18%	71%	11%
DINNER: Hot Crispy Keto Fried Chicken (page 221) and Mustard Greens with Bacon, Garlic, and Ginger (page 265)	360 70	22 6	27 2	6 7	25% 34%	68% 26%	7% 40%
OPTIONAL DESSERT: Cranberry Cherry Almond Crumble (page 295)	172	4	12	12	9%	63%	28%
SNACK: 2 hard-boiled eggs	155	13	11	1	18%	70%	12%
DAY 6 TOTAL (with dessert)	**1,389**	**76**	**100**	**43**	**22%**	**65%**	**13%**
DAY 6 TOTAL (without dessert)	**1,217**	**72**	**88**	**31**	**24%**	**65%**	**11%**
BREAKFAST: Cinnamon Roll Bites (page 158)	258	8	22	5	13%	78%	9%
LUNCH: Keto Comfort Bacon Burger (page 201)	400	26	33	6	20%	74%	6%
DINNER: Buffalo Chicken Salad (page 258)	400	19	33	8	19%	73%	8%
OPTIONAL DESSERT: Double-Chocolate Tahini Brownie (page 282)	303	7	23	17	9%	68%	23%
SNACK: Herbed Parmesan Crisps (page 189)	133	12	8	2	36%	60%	4%
DAY 7 TOTAL (with dessert)	**1,494**	**72**	**119**	**38**	**19%**	**72%**	**9%**
DAY 7 TOTAL (without dessert)	**1,191**	**65**	**96**	**21**	**21%**	**72%**	**7%**

DAY 6

DAY 7

	CALORIES	PROTEIN (G)	FAT (G)	CARBS (G)	% PROTEIN	% FAT	% CARBS
BREAKFAST: Italian-Spiced Eggs in Tomato Sauce with Ricotta (page 170)	294	16	20	14	22%	60%	18%
LUNCH: Buffalo Chicken Salad (page 258)	400	19	33	8	19%	73%	8%
DINNER: Meat Lovers' Cauliflower Pizza (page 219)	386	28	26	10	29%	61%	10%
OPTIONAL DESSERT: Chocolate Peanut Butter Fat Bombs (page 185)	122	3	12	3	9%	82%	9%
SNACK: Herbed Parmesan Crisps (page 189)	133	12	8	2	36%	60%	4%
DAY 8 TOTAL (with dessert)	**1,335**	**78**	**99**	**37**	**23%**	**67%**	**10%**
DAY 8 TOTAL (without dessert)	**1,213**	**75**	**87**	**34**	**25%**	**65%**	**10%**

DAY 8

	CALORIES	PROTEIN (G)	FAT (G)	CARBS (G)	% PROTEIN	% FAT	% CARBS
BREAKFAST: 2 hard-boiled eggs and 2 slices bacon	155 / 92	13 / 6	11 / 7	1 / 0	18% / 26%	70% / 68%	12% / 6%
LUNCH: Cajun Fish "Tacos" (page 198)	316	27	20	7	34%	57%	9%
DINNER: Sloppy Joe Pot Pie (page 232)	385	15	31	12	16%	72%	12%
OPTIONAL DESSERT: Chocolate Coconut Macadamia Ice Cream (page 287)	173	1	17	4	2%	89%	9%
SNACK: Avocado Hummus (page 181)	191	4	15	10	8%	71%	21%
DAY 9 TOTAL (with dessert)	**1,312**	**66**	**101**	**34**	**20%**	**70%**	**10%**
DAY 9 TOTAL (without dessert)	**1,139**	**65**	**84**	**30**	**24%**	**53%**	**23%**

DAY 9

	CALORIES	PROTEIN (G)	FAT (G)	CARBS (G)	% PROTEIN	% FAT	% CARBS
BREAKFAST: Grain-Free Granola (page 172)	232	5	21	7	8%	84%	8%
LUNCH: Pork Fried Rice (page 208)	360	19	24	16	22%	60%	18%
DINNER: Mushroom-Cauliflower Risotto with Pepitas (page 239)	309	15	21	15	20%	60%	20%
OPTIONAL DESSERT: Chocolate Coconut Macadamia Ice Cream (page 287)	173	1	17	4	2%	89%	9%
SNACK: 1 ounce cheddar cheese	120	6	10	0	16%	84%	0%
DAY 10 TOTAL (with dessert)	**1,194**	**46**	**93**	**42**	**15%**	**70%**	**15%**
DAY 10 TOTAL (without dessert)	**1,021**	**45**	**76**	**38**	**18%**	**67%**	**15%**

DAY 10

	CALORIES	PROTEIN (G)	FAT (G)	CARBS (G)	% PROTEIN	% FAT	% CARBS
DAY 11							
BREAKFAST: Grain-Free Granola (page 172)	232	5	21	7	8%	84%	8%
LUNCH: Classic Cobb Salad (page 254)	384	11	35	7	11%	82%	7%
DINNER: Grilled sirloin steak and Cauliflower Mashed Potatoes (page 262)	259 217	43 4	8 21	0 3	72% 7%	28% 87%	0% 6%
OPTIONAL DESSERT: Chocolate Peanut Butter Cookies (page 288)	143	6	11	5	17%	69%	14%
SNACK: 2 hard-boiled eggs	155	13	11	1	18%	70%	12%
DAY 11 TOTAL (with dessert)	**1,390**	**82**	**107**	**23**	**24%**	**69%**	**7%**
DAY 11 TOTAL (without dessert)	**1,247**	**76**	**96**	**18**	**24%**	**70%**	**6%**
DAY 12							
BREAKFAST: Egg in an Avocado with Bacon (page 169)	351	6	32	11	11%	79%	10%
LUNCH: Keto Comfort Bacon Burger (page 201)	400	26	33	6	20%	74%	6%
DINNER: Chicken and Dumpling Soup (page 243)	362	20	26	12	22%	65%	13%
OPTIONAL DESSERT: Chocolate Peanut Butter Cookies (page 288)	143	6	11	5	17%	69%	14%
SNACK: 1 ounce cheddar cheese	120	6	10	0	16%	84%	0%
DAY 12 TOTAL (with dessert)	**1,376**	**64**	**112**	**34**	**18%**	**72%**	**10%**
DAY 12 TOTAL (without dessert)	**1,233**	**58**	**101**	**29**	**18%**	**73%**	**9%**
DAY 13							
BREAKFAST: Peanut Butter Chocolate Slushee (page 137)	363	9	29	13	12%	73%	15%
LUNCH: Leftover Chicken and Dumpling Soup (page 243)	362	20	26	12	22%	65%	13%
DINNER: Grilled sirloin steak and Spicy Bacon Brussels Sprouts (page 269)	259 145	43 6	8 9	0 10	72% 16%	28% 56%	0% 28%
OPTIONAL DESSERT: Chocolate Peanut Butter Cookies (page 288)	143	6	11	5	17%	69%	14%
SNACK: Handful of almonds (25)	167	6	14	5	14%	75%	11%
DAY 13 TOTAL (with dessert)	**1,439**	**90**	**97**	**45**	**26%**	**61%**	**13%**
DAY 13 TOTAL (without dessert)	**1,296**	**84**	**86**	**40**	**27%**	**61%**	**12%**

	CALORIES	PROTEIN (G)	FAT (G)	CARBS (G)	% PROTEIN	% FAT	% CARBS
BREAKFAST: Southwestern Frittata with Chorizo (page 165)	210	11	17	3	21%	73%	6%
LUNCH: Buffalo Chicken Salad (page 258)	400	19	33	8	19%	73%	8%
DINNER: Pan-fried pork sirloin chop (boneless) and Braised Baby Bok Choy (page 273)	274 239	44 2	10 23	0 6	67% 3%	33% 87%	0% 10%
OPTIONAL DESSERT: Chocolate Chip Skillet Cookie (page 291)	262	5	22	11	8%	75%	17%
SNACK: Slice of Berry Bread with Chia Seeds (page 152)	199	6	17	9	11%	72%	17%
DAY 14 TOTAL (with dessert)	**1,584**	**87**	**122**	**37**	**22%**	**70%**	**8%**
DAY 14 TOTAL (without dessert)	**1,322**	**82**	**100**	**26**	**24%**	**68%**	**8%**

WEEK 3

	CALORIES	PROTEIN (G)	FAT (G)	CARBS (G)	% PROTEIN	% FAT	% CARBS
BREAKFAST: Mixed-Berry Smoothie (page 139)	250	14	18	6	23%	66%	11%
LUNCH: Shrimp Pad Thai (page 197)	302	29	14	17	38%	41%	21%
DINNER: Baked chicken thigh and Creamed Spinach (page 278)	296 274	37 4	15 26	0 6	54% 6%	46% 85%	0% 9%
OPTIONAL DESSERT: Chocolate Chip Skillet Cookie (page 291)	262	5	22	11	8%	75%	17%
SNACK: 1 ounce cheddar cheese	120	6	10	0	16%	84%	0%
DAY 15 TOTAL (with dessert)	**1,504**	**95**	**105**	**40**	**25%**	**63%**	**12%**
DAY 15 TOTAL (without dessert)	**1,242**	**90**	**83**	**29**	**29%**	**61%**	**10%**

	CALORIES	PROTEIN (G)	FAT (G)	CARBS (G)	% PROTEIN	% FAT	% CARBS
BREAKFAST: 2 scrambled eggs and a Lemon Poppyseed Muffin (page 156)	143 109	12 2	10 8	0 7	11% 7%	74% 66%	15% 27%
LUNCH: Herb and Garlic Salmon over Arugula (page 211)	421	26	33	6	25%	70%	5%
DINNER: Eggplant Lasagna with Beef (page 228)	385	20	27	14	22%	63%	15%
OPTIONAL DESSERT: Flourless Chocolate Cake with Almond-Coconut Cream (page 292)	292	4	24	15	6%	74%	20%
SNACK: Jalapeño Poppers with Bacon (page 186)	193	7	17	3	15%	79%	6%
DAY 16 TOTAL (with dessert)	**1,543**	**71**	**119**	**45**	**18%**	**70%**	**12%**
DAY 16 TOTAL (without dessert)	**1,251**	**67**	**95**	**30**	**22%**	**69%**	**9%**
BREAKFAST: "Hash Brown" Breakfast Bake (page 179)	331	22	24	6	27%	65%	8%
LUNCH: Chicken and Cauliflower Tikka Masala (page 212)	422	17	34	13	16%	72%	12%
DINNER: Broccoli-Cheddar Soup (page 245)	382	17	30	11	18%	71%	11%
OPTIONAL DESSERT: Chocolate Coconut Macadamia Ice Cream (page 287)	173	1	17	4	2%	89%	9%
SNACK: Jalapeño Poppers with Bacon (page 186)	193	7	17	3	15%	79%	6%
DAY 17 TOTAL (with dessert)	**1,501**	**64**	**122**	**37**	**17%**	**73%**	**10%**
DAY 17 TOTAL (without dessert)	**1,328**	**63**	**105**	**33**	**19%**	**71%**	**10%**

DAY 16

DAY 17

	CALORIES	PROTEIN (G)	FAT (G)	CARBS (G)	% PROTEIN	% FAT	% CARBS
BREAKFAST: Leftover "Hash Brown" Breakfast Bake (page 179)	331	22	24	6	27%	65%	8%
LUNCH: Steak Fajita Platter with Peppers and Avocado Mash (page 205)	395	26	27	16	25%	60%	15%
DINNER: Ground Pork Ramen (page 250)	297	11	23	12	15%	69%	16%
OPTIONAL DESSERT: Chocolate Coconut Macadamia Ice Cream (page 287)	173	1	17	4	2%	89%	9%
SNACK: Guacamole with Pepitas and Pomegranate (page 190)	195	12	14	8	23%	61%	16%
DAY 18 TOTAL (with dessert)	**1,391**	**72**	**105**	**46**	**21%**	**68%**	**11%**
DAY 18 TOTAL (without dessert)	**1,218**	**71**	**88**	**42**	**23%**	**65%**	**12%**

	CALORIES	PROTEIN (G)	FAT (G)	CARBS (G)	% PROTEIN	% FAT	% CARBS
BREAKFAST: Mixed-Berry Smoothie (page 139)	250	14	18	6	23%	66%	11%
LUNCH: Leftover Ground Pork Ramen (page 250)	297	11	23	12	15%	69%	16%
DINNER: Meat Lovers' Cauliflower Pizza (page 219)	386	28	26	10	29%	61%	10%
OPTIONAL DESSERT: Coconut Chia Blueberry Pudding (page 296)	319	5	28	13	6%	78%	16%
SNACK: Guacamole with Pepitas and Pomegranate (page 190)	195	12	14	8	23%	61%	16%
DAY 19 TOTAL (with dessert)	**1,447**	**70**	**109**	**49**	**19%**	**68%**	**13%**
DAY 19 TOTAL (without dessert)	**1,128**	**65**	**81**	**36**	**23%**	**65%**	**12%**

DAY 18

DAY 19

	CALORIES	PROTEIN (G)	FAT (G)	CARBS (G)	% PROTEIN	% FAT	% CARBS
BREAKFAST: Grain-Free Granola (page 172)	232	5	21	7	8%	84%	8%
LUNCH: Mediterranean Salmon Burger (page 202)	371	34	23	7	36%	56%	8%
DINNER: Grilled sirloin steak and Cauliflower Mashed Potatoes (page 262)	259 217	43 4	8 21	0 3	72% 7%	28% 87%	0% 6%
OPTIONAL DESSERT: Coconut Chia Blueberry Pudding (page 296)	319	5	28	13	6%	78%	16%
SNACK: 2 hard-boiled eggs	155	13	11	1	18%	70%	12%
DAY 20 TOTAL (with dessert)	**1,553**	**104**	**112**	**31**	**27%**	**65%**	**8%**
DAY 20 TOTAL (without dessert)	**1,234**	**99**	**84**	**18**	**33%**	**61%**	**6%**
BREAKFAST: 2 scrambled eggs and a slice of Chocolate Zucchini Bread (page 161)	155 353	13 9	11 29	1 14	18% 10%	70% 74%	12% 16%
LUNCH: Kale and Spinach Caesar Salad (page 253)	315	8	29	5	10%	84%	6%
DINNER: The Ultimate Meatloaf (page 236)	361	22	29	3	25%	72%	3%
OPTIONAL DESSERT: Coconut Chia Blueberry Pudding (page 296)	319	5	28	13	6%	78%	16%
SNACK: 1 ounce cheddar cheese	120	6	10	0	16%	84%	0%
DAY 21 TOTAL (with dessert)	**1,623**	**63**	**136**	**36**	**16%**	**75%**	**9%**
DAY 21 TOTAL (without dessert)	**1,304**	**58**	**108**	**23**	**18%**	**75%**	**7%**

DAY 20

DAY 21

PERSONALIZE YOUR DAILY MEALS

When not using recipes, create "throw-together" meals such as those I described in the previous chapter (page 104), and intersperse them in your plan.

BREAKFAST

On Tier 3, you'll be eating breakfast, which is structured like this: a protein + fat + nonstarchy vegetables or a keto-friendly fruit (optional + keto comfort food bread or pastry). For example:

Eggs + bacon, sausage, or ham + a bowl of fresh berries

Cheese omelet made with veggies like spinach, tomatoes, and mushrooms

Grain-free granola + almond milk

Keto comfort food slushee or smoothie (pages 137 to 144)

LUNCH, DINNER, AND SNACKS

Follow the suggestions for Tier 2 on page 103.

To assist you in planning your meals on Tier 3, here is a daily worksheet that can be copied as needed and filled in.

MEAL-PLANNING WORKSHEET

BREAKFAST

_____ OR _____
KETO COMFORT FOOD BREAKFAST RECIPE — PROTEIN

OR _____ — FAT
└ KETO COMFORT FOOD SMOOTHIE OR SLUSHEE RECIPE

└ OPTIONAL NONSTARCHY VEGETABLES
OR KETO-FRIENDLY FRUIT

└ OPTIONAL KETO COMFORT FOOD BREAD
OR PASTRY RECIPE

LUNCH

_____ OR _____
KETO COMFORT FOOD LUNCH RECIPE — PROTEIN

OR _____ — NONSTARCHY VEGETABLES
└ KETO COMFORT FOOD SALAD, SOUP, OR STEW RECIPE

└ FAT

DINNER

_____
KETO COMFORT FOOD DINNER RECIPE

OR _____
├ PROTEIN

├ NONSTARCHY VEGETABLES OR KETO COMFORT
FOOD SIDE RECIPE

├ FAT

└ OPTIONAL KETO COMFORT FOOD DESSERT RECIPE

SNACK

_____
KETO COMFORT FOOD SNACK RECIPE

OR _____
└ SNACK FROM THE APPROVED LIST (SEE PAGE 103)

MY DAILY NUTRITION

_____
TOTAL CALORIES

_____
TOTAL GRAMS OF PROTEIN

_____
TOTAL GRAMS OF FAT

_____
TOTAL GRAMS OF CARBOHYDRATES

_____
DAILY PERCENTAGE OF PROTEIN

_____
DAILY PERCENTAGE OF FAT

_____
DAILY PERCENTAGE OF CARBOHYDRATES

Watch your portions when planning meals. The recipes are portion controlled for you, so you don't have to worry about measuring things out. The portion sizes of my recipes can also teach key lessons, like what a single portion of protein or veggies really should look like.

TIER 3 GUIDELINES

Up to now, you have probably been burning fat at the speed of light, or close to it. On this tier, your weight loss may slow down a bit—but don't get discouraged. You should still be in ketosis, and your body by now is most likely fat-adapted, so you're burning fat naturally. The goal of this tier is to cement new eating habits and produce steady, satisfying weight loss.

1. Follow Tier 3 for 21 days. If you have more weight to lose, you can stay on Tier 3 or accelerate your weight loss by going back to Tier 2.

2. With the addition of optional desserts, your carb count may inch up near 50 grams that day. But by skipping dessert, your carb count will be around 40 grams a day or lower. The menus show how desserts fit into the plan, but you do not have to have a dessert every day (even though they are delicious!).

3. Include protein, nonstarchy veggies, and fat at each main meal.

4. As for intermittent fasting, if you enjoyed that strategy and found it effective and doable, it is fine to continue it for several days a week.

5. If you have found recipes that you and your family really love, feel free to enjoy them on multiple days.

6. Avoid sugary and high-starch foods completely, as well as junk foods, processed foods, and low-fat foods.

7. Stay well hydrated.

8. You may enjoy alcohol occasionally, but in moderation—around 3 drinks a week. If drinking alcohol affects your ketosis negatively, avoid it.

9. Review the shopping lists in Appendix A prior to going to the grocery store.

10. Choose organic for both produce and animal products if possible.

11. Study the recipes carefully prior to cooking them. They are easy to prepare.

12. Test yourself daily (in the morning and afternoon) to make sure you're staying in ketosis. Keep track of your weight loss every few days.

TIER 4: KETO COMFORT PHASING

Standing ovation . . . applause! Congratulations are in order: You've hit your ideal weight and your body is more contoured than ever because you've lost inches of pure fat.

Now what? How do you keep your lean, healthier physique?

Here's where the maintenance part of the Keto Comfort Food Diet comes into play: Keto Comfort Phasing, or KCP for short. It is actually a less-restrictive form of keto dieting (Yes, more carbs. Yippee!) that helps you stay trim and fit.

And it is great for successful maintenance. At least one analysis of keto diets found that they are associated with better weight maintenance over time, even after the diet ended and people returned to their normal eating patterns.

KCP means following 4 to 5 days of keto comfort food dieting (usually during weekdays) and then higher-carb days on the weekend. In other words, you eat ketogenically through the week and allow yourself more leeway on the weekend. This cycles your body in and out of ketosis and is beneficial for overall health and energy.

Why did I structure it like this? Let's face it, weekends have never been kind to the waistline. There's TGIF with friends . . . parties on Saturdays . . . Sunday dinners with family . . . basically lots of socializing that can do you in. We're happy to toss our diets out the window and promise to get back on course on Monday. It just makes sense that this is a great way to structure a maintenance plan. You can still eat ketogenically during the week, using your favorite keto comfort food recipes, then on weekends have a more varied diet.

KCP is not a free-for-all, however. You can reintroduce a lot of your favorite carb foods (if you want to), but only in moderation. No pig-outs! In other words, be a little more liberal in eating carbs to have with one or two of your favorite meals.

HOW TO START KCP

This maintenance plan is unique because it helps you keep your weight off, while allowing you to eat a wider range of foods two to three times a week.

TO REITERATE

Monday breakfast through Friday lunch (or dinner), follow the Keto Comfort Food Diet meal plans, either Tier 2 (Acceleration) or Tier 3 (Basic), incorporating your favorite recipes from this book. Stick to 20 to 40 grams of carbs daily.

Phase in higher-carb eating on the weekends. The weight loss you've achieved will correct any insulin resistance and thus improve your metabolism to handle additional carbohydrates. But if the scale starts creeping up, along with your carb intake, ease back and find a daily carb level that reduces and stabilizes your weight.

KETO COMFORT PHASING—A 7-DAY SAMPLE MEAL PLAN FOR MAINTENANCE

Here is a 7-day sample of how to structure your meals in maintenance, along with recipes, calorie counts, and macro percentages.

		CALORIES	PROTEIN (G)	FAT (G)	CARBS (G)	% PROTEIN	% FAT	% CARBS
MONDAY	Black coffee, green tea, or lemon water	-	-	-	-	-	-	-
	LUNCH: Keto Comfort Bacon Burger (page 201)	400	26	33	6	20%	74%	6%
	DINNER: Nut-Crusted Fish (page 235) with The Creamiest Coleslaw with Dill (page 257)	344 246	38 2	20 22	3 10	44% 3%	52% 81%	4% 16%
	SNACK: Chocolate Peanut Butter Fat Bombs (page 185)	122	3	12	3	9%	82%	9%
	MONDAY TOTAL	**1,112**	**69**	**87**	**22**	**24%**	**70%**	**6%**
TUESDAY	Black coffee, green tea, or lemon water	-	-	-	-	-	-	-
	LUNCH: Cajun Fish "Tacos" (page 198)	316	27	20	7	34%	57%	9%
	DINNER: Sloppy Joe Pot Pie (page 232)	385	15	31	12	16%	72%	12%
	OPTIONAL DESSERT: Chocolate Coconut Macadamia Ice Cream (page 287)	173	1	17	4	2%	89%	9%
	SNACK: Spinach and Artichoke Dip (page 192)	284	9	24	8	13%	76%	11%
	TUESDAY TOTAL (including dessert)	**1,158**	**52**	**92**	**31**	**18%**	**72%**	**10%**
WEDNESDAY	**BREAKFAST:** Blueberry Pancakes (page 166)	418	12	33	20	11%	70%	19%
	LUNCH: Classic Cobb Salad (page 254)	384	11	35	7	11%	82%	7%
	DINNER: The Ultimate Meatloaf (page 236)	361	22	29	3	25%	72%	3%
	SNACK: Leftover Spinach and Artichoke Dip (page 192)	284	9	24	8	13%	76%	11%
	WEDNESDAY TOTAL	**1,447**	**54**	**121**	**38**	**15%**	**75%**	**10%**

	CALORIES	PROTEIN (G)	FAT (G)	CARBS (G)	% PROTEIN	% FAT	% CARBS
BREAKFAST: Southwestern Frittata with Chorizo (page 165)	210	11	17	3	21%	73%	6%
LUNCH: Leftover The Ultimate Meatloaf (page 236)	361	22	29	3	25%	72%	3%
DINNER: Shrimp and Cheesy Cauliflower Grits (page 226)	316	34	17	6	43%	49%	8%
OPTIONAL DESSERT: Ricotta Cheesecake with Strawberry Sauce (page 283)	351	12	31	6	14%	79%	7%
SNACK: Cauliflower Hummus (page 182)	255	5	21	12	7%	75%	18%
THURSDAY TOTAL (including dessert)	**1,493**	**84**	**115**	**30**	**22%**	**70%**	**8%**
BREAKFAST: Chocolate-Glazed Doughnut (page 157)	241	4	21	9	7%	78%	15%
LUNCH: Tuna Salad over Bibb (page 204)	393	37	23	4	38%	53%	9%
DINNER: Grilled sirloin steak,	259	43	8	0	72%	28%	0%
medium baked potato, and Green Beans	168	5	0	37	12%	0%	88%
in Garlic Sauce (page 277)	287	4	23	16	6%	72%	22%
SNACK: Handful of almonds (25)	167	6	14	5	14%	75%	11%
FRIDAY TOTAL	**1,515**	**99**	**89**	**71**	**26%**	**54%**	**20%**
BREAKFAST: 1 cup oatmeal,	150	5	3	27	13%	18%	69%
½ cup strawberries, and	27	0	0	6	0%	0%	100%
½ cup almond milk	15	0	0	0	0%	0%	0%
LUNCH: Texas-Style Chili (page 249)	366	16	25	20	17%	61%	22%
DINNER AT AN ASIAN RESTAURANT:							
Cashew chicken stir fry,	580	32	35	32	22%	54%	24%
½ cup brown rice, and	109	2	0	23	7%	0%	93%
two 5-ounce glasses white wine	242	0	0	3	0%	0%	100%
SNACK: 1 ounce cheddar cheese	120	6	10	0	16%	84%	0%
SATURDAY TOTAL	**1,609**	**61**	**73**	**111**	**16%**	**41%**	**43%***

*includes 15% alcohol

THURSDAY

FRIDAY

SATURDAY

	CALORIES	PROTEIN (G)	FAT (G)	CARBS (G)	% PROTEIN	% FAT	% CARBS
BREAKFAST: Chocolate Chip Waffles (page 176)	369	13	32	11	11%	74%	15%
LUNCH: Leftover Texas-Style Chili (page 249)	366	16	25	20	17%	61%	22%
DINNER: Hot Crispy Keto Fried Chicken (page 221) and a baked medium sweet potato	360 100	22 2	27 0	6 23	25% 8%	68% 0%	7% 92%
OPTIONAL DESSERT: Chocolate Avocado Mousse (page 280)	218	3	18	11	6%	74%	20%
SNACK: 1 medium apple	93	1	0	25	4%	0%	96%
SUNDAY TOTAL (including dessert)	**1,506**	**57**	**102**	**96**	**15%**	**61%**	**24%**

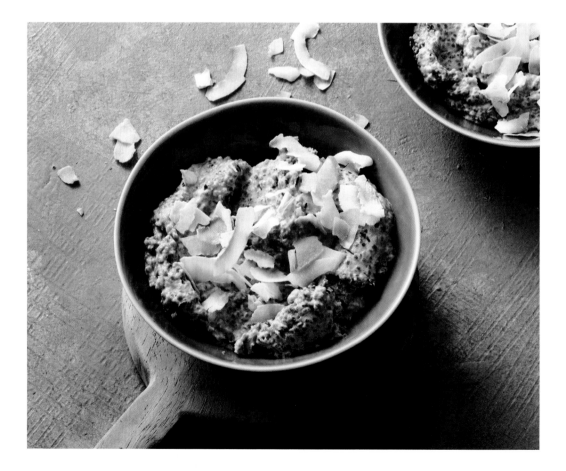

To assist you in planning your meals on KCP, here is a daily worksheet that can be copied as needed and filled in.

BREAKFAST

_____

⌐ PROTEIN
+
⊢ FAT
+
⊢ OPTIONAL NONSTARCHY VEGETABLES
   OR KETO-FRIENDLY FRUIT
+
⌐ OPTIONAL KETO COMFORT FOOD BREAD
⌐ OR PASTRY RECIPE

OR _____
⌐ KETO COMFORT FOOD BREAKFAST RECIPE

OR _____
⌐ KETO COMFORT FOOD SMOOTHIE OR SLUSHEE RECIPE

LUNCH

_____

KETO COMFORT FOOD LUNCH RECIPE

OR _____
⌐ KETO COMFORT FOOD SALAD, SOUP,
   OR STEW RECIPE

OR _____
⊢ PROTEIN
+
⊢ NONSTARCHY VEGETABLES
+
⊢ STARCHY CARBOHYDRATE
+
⌐ FAT

DINNER

_____

KETO COMFORT FOOD DINNER RECIPE

OR _____
⊢ PROTEIN
+
⊢ NONSTARCHY VEGETABLES
+
⊢ STARCHY CARBOHYDRATE
+
⊢ FAT
+
⌐ OPTIONAL KETO COMFORT FOOD DESSERT RECIPE

MY DAILY NUTRITION

_____

TOTAL CALORIES

_____

TOTAL GRAMS OF PROTEIN

_____

TOTAL GRAMS OF FAT

_____

TOTAL GRAMS OF CARBOHYDRATES

_____

DAILY PERCENTAGE OF PROTEIN

_____

DAILY PERCENTAGE OF FAT

_____

DAILY PERCENTAGE OF CARBOHYDRATES

SNACK

_____

KETO COMFORT FOOD SNACK RECIPE

OR _____
⌐ SNACK FROM THE APPROVED LIST

OR _____
⌐ FRESH FRUIT SERVING

Watch your portions when planning meals. The recipes are portion controlled for you, so you don't have to worry about measuring things out. The portion sizes of my recipes can also teach key lessons, like what a single portion of protein or veggies really should look like.

OTHER IMPORTANT GUIDELINES FOR SUCCESS ON MAINTENANCE

1. **Choose your extra carbs wisely.** They should come from "clean sources": oatmeal, brown rice, quinoa, legumes, whole-grain or legume-based pasta, whole-grain bread, winter squashes, root vegetables (potato, sweet potato, turnips, carrots, beets, parsnips, and so on). Avoid highly processed foods. Allow yourself 1 portion daily, if desired. Portions are:

Baked potato, sweet potato, or beet: 1 medium (meaning it can fit in your cupped hand)

Other starchy vegetables: ½ cup mashed turnips or parsnips; 2 carrots (raw) or ½ cup cooked; ½ cup cooked corn or peas

Legumes or lentils: ½ cup

Winter squash: 1 cup

Pasta (whole-grain): ½ cup

Brown rice, cooked: ½ cup

Quinoa, cooked: ½ cup

Oats or other cooked cereal: ½ cup

Cold cereal, unsweetened: 1 cup

Bread: 1 or 2 slices

Bun (hamburger size) or roll (2 inches square): 1

Crackers (whole-grain): 4 to 6

2. **Incorporate carb "swaps."** If you find that eating these carbs is triggering weight gain, cut back and swap them out for these keto substitutes:

STARCHY CARBOHYDRATES	KETO SWAPS
Bread	Lettuce leaves, portobello mushrooms
Bread crumbs	Crushed pork rinds, almond flour, Parmesan crisps, or crushed nuts
Cereal, granola	Grain-Free Granola (page 172)
Flour	Almond flour, coconut flour
French fries	Zucchini fries
Pasta	Zoodles (zucchini noodles), butternut squash fettuccine, eggplant sliced into lasagna-like "noodles," spaghetti squash, shirataki noodles

Pizza	Cauliflower pizza
Potato	Mashed cauliflower
Potato chips	Kale chips, cheese crisps
Rice	Cauliflower rice, shirataki rice
Tortillas	Lettuce leaves, coconut wraps

3. **Make reintroduced carbs the accent for meals—not the centerpiece.** Enjoy your carbs but don't eat ginormous mounds of pasta or rice or other starchy foods for dinner. Keep the emphasis on protein and some healthy fats.

4. **Expand your fruit choices, but don't go overboard.** Have only 1 to 2 servings a day of carbs or fruit. A serving size for women is ½ cup; for men, 1 cup. Continue to watch your portion sizes; adhering to them can significantly help with weight management.

5. **Discourage weekend carbs from being stored as fat.** For example, eat them just prior to or right after a workout. And no carbs close to bedtime!

6. **On the higher-carb days (weekends), decrease your fats.** As you've learned, fats on the Keto Comfort Food Diet are important because they support ketosis, add flavor to foods, curb appetite control, and make the plan sustainable in the long run. However, when you bring some carbs back, your fats need to go down; otherwise, you'll be taking in too many calories. So don't be overgenerous with fats.

7. **Eat some greens daily.** Leafy green veggies are a fantastic source of fiber, iron, calcium, folate, potassium, vitamins A, C, and K—need I continue? Add kale, spinach, and broccoli to smoothies to get your fix.

8. **Eat whole, unprocessed organic food.** Organic food is very important to me, and it's important to your ongoing health. I'm strict about it; heck, I'm practically militant about it. I'm part of the segment of people in this country who eat organic food and consider it something of a religion. I think it tastes better. It's nutritionally more valuable. I believe there's a connection between bad health and the chemicals present in nonorganic food. I get very distressed about fast food, genetically modified food, junk food, and processed food. My own pantry proves how dedicated I am to the cause; it's filled with organic staples of all kinds. When you eat real food—organic food—it will be easier to keep your weight off. It is more satisfying and filling than processed food. Most of the time, it's lower in calories and carbs and will help to naturally keep you in great shape.

9. **Have one "favorite food" meal during the week, or preferably on the weekend.** This could be one or two slices of pizza, a steak and baked potato, or some enchiladas. And finish off with a dessert.

10. **Don't go back to your former eating habits!** The way you ate in the past put on weight, made you unhealthy, and probably made you very unhappy. That's what got you into trouble in the first place, and you don't want to mess up your metabolism and health again. Be good to your body! That said, if you succumb to those bad habits, get back on the Keto Comfort Food Diet. Or periodically go to Tier 1, the 3-Day Keto Cleanse. It's a great tool—one you can call upon if diet disaster hits!

11. **Weigh yourself frequently.** Have a weight range you consider acceptable—I recommend 3 pounds. If you exceed that range, go back on the plan until you return to your ideal weight. Always monitor your weight!

12. **Don't forget to hydrate.** On KCP, it's key to drink plenty of water throughout the day. Liquids help keep food moving along through your digestive system, hydrate cells from the inside so that your whole body benefits, and tame hunger even more by keeping your stomach partially filled.

13. **Do intermittent fasting periodically during the week.** It is a powerful maintenance tool. I typically fast two to three times a week.

14. **Make a lifetime commitment to exercise.** Studies show that people who lose weight and keep it off work out on a regular basis. Their activity averages an hour a day. Resistance training, which builds and preserves fat-burning muscle, is one of the best activities for weight maintenance, especially if you practice intermittent fasting.

If you have been successful on my Keto Comfort Food Diet, you have cemented some great nutritional habits—like eating more vegetables, moving away from too many carbs, breaking a sugar addiction, and developing a healthier relationship with food. You've learned how to make super delicious foods, while your body has learned to energize itself from ketone bodies and fat.

All of these lessons will help you for the rest of your life, as long as you continue to practice them!

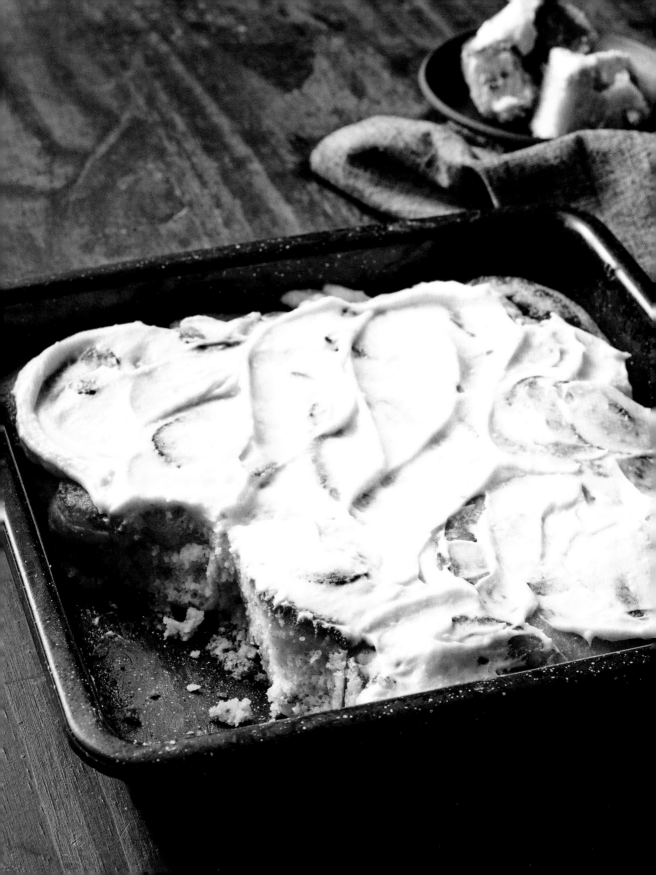

PART THREE

THE KETO COMFORT FOOD RECIPES

SMOOTHIES + BEVERAGES

We all lead insanely hectic lives at times—which is why I like quick beverages like smoothies for breakfast and snacks. Anyone can make them in a matter of minutes. In one glass, you get all the nutrition you need for the morning. What could be simpler?

Many smoothies in stores and restaurants contain large amounts of sugar. I make mine high in water and fiber, and often fortify them with a protein powder.

Also included here is my version of the ever-popular keto coffee, designed to help the body get into ketosis. It's quick and easy to prepare, too.

Finally, enjoy my keto "kocktails" when you get to Tiers 3 and 4.

KETO BREAKFAST COFFEE

PREP TIME: 5 MINUTES ★ SERVINGS: 1

Here's a real kick-start into ketosis—a cup of frothy deliciousness
with fat-burning fats to begin your day. This recipe is your morning
routine on my 3-Day Keto Cleanse. Use it beyond the cleanse, too.
Caffeinated beverages, including coffee, have recently been shown
in research to support weight-loss maintenance.

1 cup of your favorite hot
coffee

1 teaspoon ghee

1 tablespoon MCT oil

¼ teaspoon ground cinnamon

¼ teaspoon vanilla extract

1 to 2 tablespoons granulated
erythritol (optional)

In a blender, combine all the ingredients and blend until
frothy and smooth.

PER SERVING ★ CALORIES: 161 ★ GRAMS OF PROTEIN: 0 ★ GRAMS OF FAT: 19 ★ GRAMS OF CARBOHYDRATE: 0
★ PERCENT OF PROTEIN: 0% ★ PERCENT OF FAT: 100% ★ PERCENT OF CARBOHYDRATE: 0%

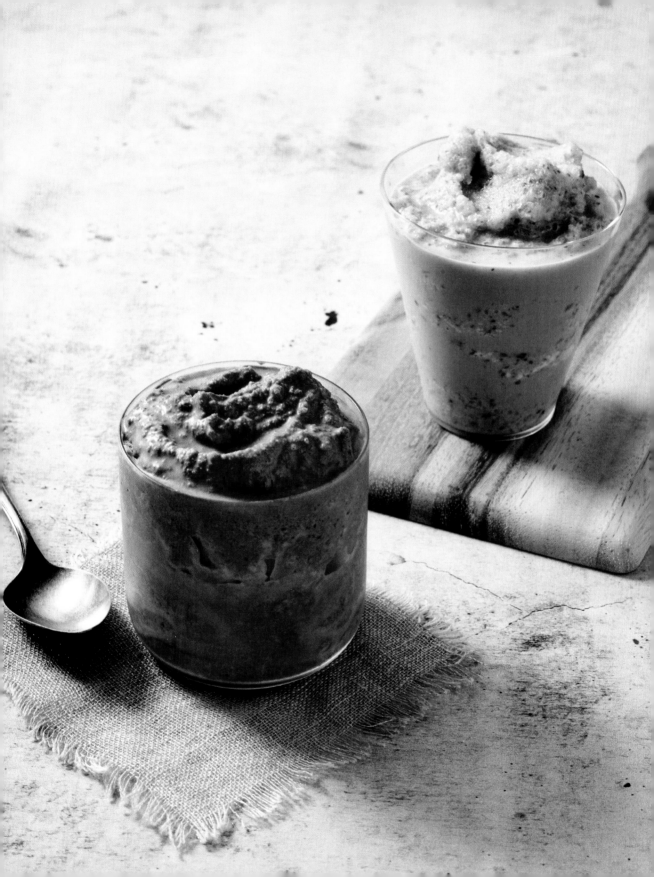

PEANUT BUTTER CHOCOLATE SLUSHEE

PREP TIME: 5 MINUTES ★ SERVINGS: 1

Here's an icy treat that's like sipping a candy bar of chocolate and peanut butter—a quick breakfast drink for any morning of the week.

2 tablespoons + 2 teaspoons full-fat unsweetened coconut milk, chilled

2 tablespoons heavy cream, chilled

¼ teaspoon vanilla extract

1½ tablespoons unsweetened cocoa powder

1 tablespoon + ¾ teaspoon granulated erythritol

1½ tablespoons creamy unsweetened natural peanut butter

½ cup crushed ice

In a blender, combine all the ingredients and blend until smooth.

PER SERVING ★ CALORIES: 363 ★ GRAMS OF PROTEIN: 9 ★ GRAMS OF FAT: 29 ★ GRAMS OF CARBOHYDRATE: 13 ★ PERCENT OF PROTEIN: 12% ★ PERCENT OF FAT: 73% ★ PERCENT OF CARBOHYDRATE: 15%

SPINACH-CANTALOUPE SLUSHEE

PREP TIME: 5 MINUTES ★ SERVINGS: 1

Two powerhouse plant foods—spinach and cantaloupe—cuddle up here for a refreshing, nutrient-packed treat.

¼ cup cantaloupe chunks, frozen

¼ cup baby spinach

¼ cup whole milk

¼ cup water

½ scoop vanilla protein powder (such as Isopure)

1½ teaspoons granulated erythritol

1½ teaspoons fresh lemon juice

1 tablespoon MCT oil

¼ cup crushed ice

In a blender, combine all the ingredients and blend until smooth.

PER SERVING ★ CALORIES: 304 ★ GRAMS OF PROTEIN: 18 ★ GRAMS OF FAT: 20 ★ GRAMS OF CARBOHYDRATE: 12 ★ PERCENT OF PROTEIN: 24% ★ PERCENT OF FAT: 60% ★ PERCENT OF CARBOHYDRATE: 16%

MIXED-BERRY SMOOTHIE

PREP TIME: 5 MINUTES ★ SERVINGS: 1

Berries are your best keto bet for fruit because they're low in sugar.
They also pair well with greens like kale in smoothies.

¼ cup frozen mixed berries, such as blueberries and raspberries

¼ cup baby kale

¼ cup water

¼ cup crushed ice

½ scoop vanilla protein powder (such as Isopure)

½ tablespoon almond butter

1 tablespoon granulated erythritol (optional)

1 tablespoon MCT oil

In a blender, combine all the ingredients and blend until smooth.

PER SERVING ★ CALORIES: 250 ★ GRAMS OF PROTEIN: 14 ★ GRAMS OF FAT: 18 ★ GRAMS OF CARBOHYDRATE: 6 ★ PERCENT OF PROTEIN: 23% ★ PERCENT OF FAT: 66% ★ PERCENT OF CARBOHYDRATE: 11%

COCONUT-STRAWBERRY SMOOTHIE

GREEN AVOCADO SMOOTHIE

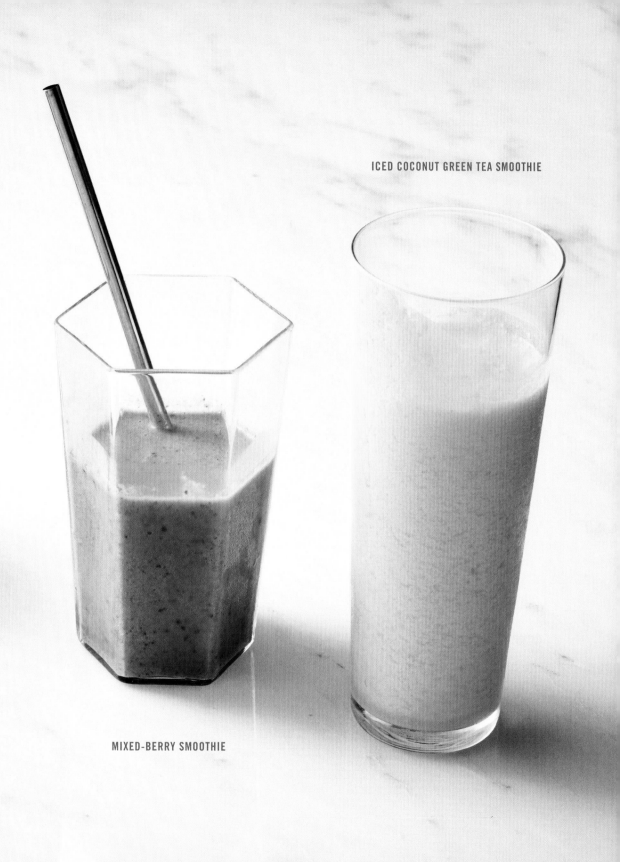

ICED COCONUT GREEN TEA SMOOTHIE

MIXED-BERRY SMOOTHIE

GREEN AVOCADO SMOOTHIE

PREP TIME: 5 MINUTES ★ SERVINGS: 1

This glass of delight has avocado for added richness. Avocado is technically a fruit—one that contains heart-healthy monounsaturated fats, which can lower cholesterol levels.

½ avocado, halved and pitted

½ cup well-packed baby kale

¾ cup water

½ cup crushed ice

2 tablespoons granulated erythritol (optional)

2 tablespoons fresh lemon juice

1 tablespoon MCT oil

Scoop the avocado flesh into a blender. Add the remaining ingredients and blend until smooth.

TIP: Blend smoothies for at least 5 minutes. This pumps up the recipe with extra air, which will make you feel full.

PER SERVING ★ CALORIES: 308 ★ GRAMS OF PROTEIN: 3 ★ GRAMS OF FAT: 29 ★ GRAMS OF CARBOHYDRATE: 15 ★ PERCENT OF PROTEIN: 4% ★ PERCENT OF FAT: 81% ★ PERCENT OF CARBOHYDRATE: 15%

COCONUT-STRAWBERRY SMOOTHIE

PREP TIME: 5 MINUTES ★ SERVINGS: 1

This smoothie is one of my favorites. It's souped up with high-antioxidant strawberries and fat-burning MCT oil. All the coconut extras give it a tropical taste.

¼ cup frozen strawberries

2 tablespoons + 2 teaspoons full-fat unsweetened coconut milk, chilled

2 tablespoons water

¼ cup crushed ice

¼ teaspoon coconut extract

1 tablespoon granulated erythritol

½ tablespoon chia seeds

½ scoop vanilla protein powder (such as Isopure)

1 tablespoon MCT oil

In a blender, combine all the ingredients and blend until smooth. Add more water if needed.

PER SERVING ★ CALORIES: 327 ★ GRAMS OF PROTEIN: 6 ★ GRAMS OF FAT: 28 ★ GRAMS OF CARBOHYDRATE: 10 ★ PERCENT OF PROTEIN: 9% ★ PERCENT OF FAT: 78% ★ PERCENT OF CARBOHYDRATE: 13%

ICED COCONUT GREEN TEA SMOOTHIE

PREP TIME: 5 MINUTES ★ SERVINGS: 1

Green tea is well known for its fat-burning dividend. Add to it fresh ginger and turmeric, two spices that are full of phytochemicals that fight inflammation, and you've got an irresistible taste combination.

¾ cup unsweetened brewed green tea, chilled

½ cup full-fat unsweetened coconut milk, chilled

1 tablespoon fresh lemon juice

1 tablespoon grated peeled fresh ginger

2 teaspoons grated peeled fresh turmeric

2 tablespoons granulated erythritol

1 tablespoon MCT oil

1 cup crushed ice

In a blender, combine all the ingredients and blend until smooth.

PER SERVING ★ CALORIES: 377 ★ GRAMS OF PROTEIN: 2 ★ GRAMS OF FAT: 37 ★ GRAMS OF CARBOHYDRATE: 12 ★ PERCENT OF PROTEIN: 2% ★ PERCENT OF FAT: 86% ★ PERCENT OF CARBOHYDRATE: 12%

CUCUMBER-MINT MOJITO WITH VODKA

PREP TIME: 5 MINUTES ★ SERVINGS: 2

The name of this world-famous cocktail derives from *mojo*, an African word meaning to cast a spell. There is something magical about this drink for sure. It tastes delicious in the heat of summer, and writer Ernest Hemingway was a big fan. I've cast a new spell on it by making it with vodka rather than rum, and adding cucumber to the mix.

4 slices English cucumber

¼ cup fresh mint leaves, plus 2 sprigs for garnish

3 to 4 tablespoons granulated erythritol, to taste

2 tablespoons fresh lime juice

3 ounces vodka

Sparkling water

2 lime wheels, for garnish

Muddle the cucumber, mint leaves, and erythritol in the bottom of a cocktail shaker. Add some ice, the lime juice, and vodka and shake until cold and lightly frothy. Strain into two tall ice-filled glasses and top with sparkling water. Garnish each with a lime wheel and a mint sprig.

PER SERVING ★ CALORIES: 106 ★ GRAMS OF PROTEIN: 0 ★ GRAMS OF FAT: 0 ★ GRAMS OF CARBOHYDRATE: 3 ★ PERCENT OF PROTEIN: 0% ★ PERCENT OF FAT: 0% ★ PERCENT OF CARBOHYDRATE: 100%

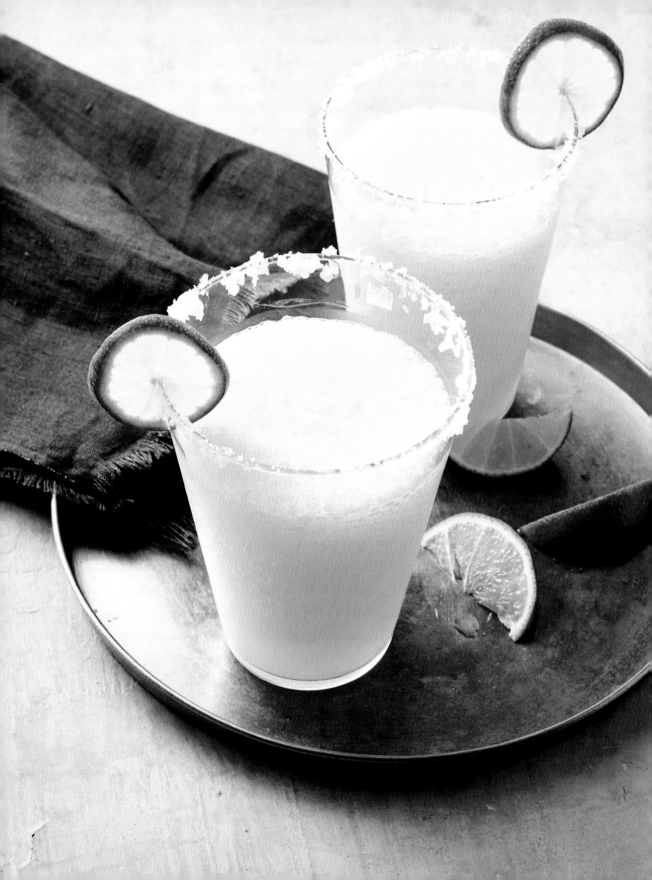

FROZEN KETO MARGARITA

PREP TIME: 5 MINUTES ★ SERVINGS: 2

Did you know that a lot of margaritas may contain up to 900 calories a serving? Not this one! You can enjoy a little alcohol on this diet, but don't overdo it. Too much alcohol interferes with the liver's ability to burn fat.

½ cup blanco tequila

½ cup fresh lime juice, plus more for rimming the glass

¼ cup fresh lemon juice

¼ cup fresh orange juice

2½ cups crushed ice

2 tablespoons granulated erythritol

Celtic sea salt, for rimming

2 lime wheels, for garnish

In a blender, combine the tequila, fruit juices, ice, and erythritol and blend until smooth. Dip the rim of two glasses in lime juice, then in sea salt. Pour in the margaritas and garnish each drink with a lime wheel.

PER SERVING ★ CALORIES: 48 ★ GRAMS OF PROTEIN: 1 ★ GRAMS OF FAT: 0 ★ GRAMS OF CARBOHYDRATE: 11 ★ PERCENT OF PROTEIN: 8% ★ PERCENT OF FAT: 0% ★ PERCENT OF CARBOHYDRATE: 92%

KETO BLOODY MARY

PREP TIME: 5 MINUTES ★ SERVINGS: 2

This classic cocktail was created at a New York City bar in 1934 and has been a favorite ever since. I like mine spicy like this one. Leave out the vodka and you have a Virgin Mary.

½ cup tomato juice

½ cup vodka

1½ teaspoons coconut aminos

1 teaspoon horseradish

2 tablespoons fresh lemon juice

Celtic sea salt

Freshly ground black pepper

Hot sauce

2 celery sticks, for garnish

2 lemon wedges, for garnish

6 pimiento-stuffed olives, for garnish

Combine the tomato juice, vodka, coconut aminos, horseradish, lemon juice, and sea salt, black pepper, and hot sauce to taste in a cocktail shaker. Shake to combine. Divide between two ice-filled glasses and garnish each with a celery stick, a lemon wedge, and 3 olives threaded with a toothpick.

PER SERVING ★ CALORIES: 76 ★ GRAMS OF PROTEIN: 1 ★ GRAMS OF FAT: 4 ★ GRAMS OF CARBOHYDRATE: 9 ★ PERCENT OF PROTEIN: 5% ★ PERCENT OF FAT: 48% ★ PERCENT OF CARBOHYDRATE: 47%

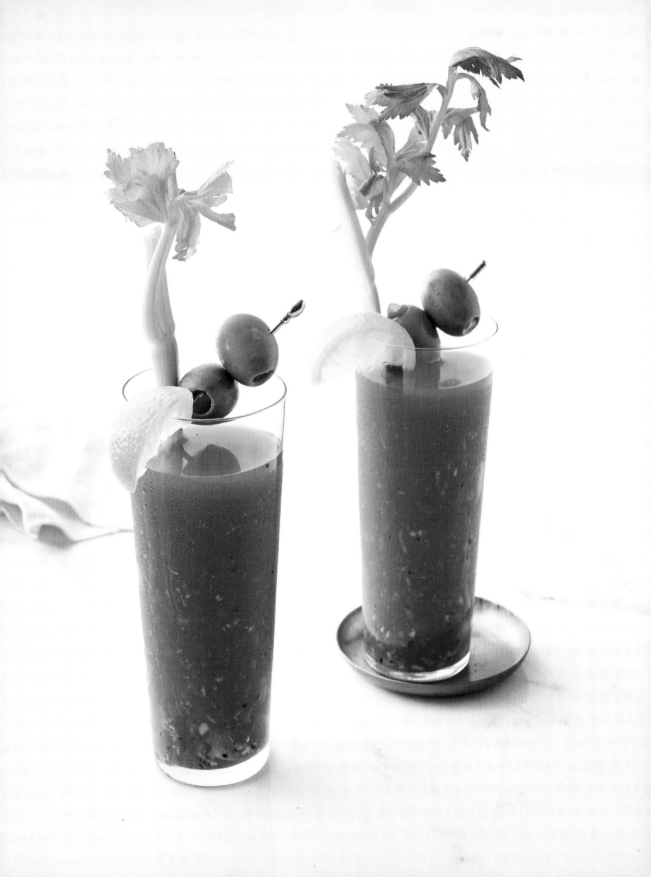

BREADS + PASTRIES

Bread? Pastries? On a keto diet? Who am I kidding?

No one!

I love fluffy bread or a sweet pastry as much as the next person, but when keto dieting, we have to deny ourselves. So I spent a lot of time removing the carbs from breads, pastries, muffins, and more—so that we can all indulge again. The trick is using low-carb flours (which are healthier for you anyway because they're gluten-free).

With most of these recipes, I like to whip up a batch ahead of time and pair a serving with scrambled eggs or some Greek yogurt for a quick, complete breakfast. Or enjoy them as a snack. My Keto Dinner Rolls and Cheddar and Chive Biscuits return bread to your evening meal.

Bread is back!

SEEDED TAHINI BREAD

PREP TIME: 10 MINUTES ★ COOK TIME: 35 MINUTES ★ SERVINGS: 8

Tahini is sesame seed butter, usually reserved for making hummus. I've found it makes a great-tasting base for keto bread. I love a slice of this bread in the morning, slathered with almond butter.

Coconut oil, melted, for the pan

1 cup tahini

4 large eggs

1 tablespoon fresh lemon juice

1 teaspoon baking soda

2 tablespoons ground flaxseeds

1½ tablespoons chia seeds

½ teaspoon Celtic sea salt

2 tablespoons granulated erythritol

4 tablespoons hulled pumpkin seeds (pepitas), toasted

1 tablespoon sesame seeds, toasted

1. Preheat the oven to 350°F. Grease a 9 x 5-inch loaf pan with coconut oil and line with parchment paper, going up two sides of the pan.

2. In a large bowl, whisk together the tahini, eggs, and lemon juice until combined. Add the baking soda, flaxseeds, chia seeds, sea salt, erythritol, and 3 tablespoons of the pumpkin seeds. Stir until combined.

3. Scrape the batter into the prepared pan, smooth the top, and sprinkle with the sesame seeds and the remaining 1 tablespoon pumpkin seeds. Bake until an inserted toothpick comes out clean, 30 to 35 minutes. Cover the bread with foil if it starts to get too dark while baking. Allow to cool for 10 minutes in the pan, then remove to a wire rack to cool completely. Slice and serve.

PER SERVING ★ CALORIES: 282 ★ GRAMS OF PROTEIN: 10 ★ GRAMS OF FAT: 22 ★ GRAMS OF CARBOHYDRATE: 11 ★ PERCENT OF PROTEIN: 15% ★ PERCENT OF FAT: 70% ★ PERCENT OF CARBOHYDRATE: 15%

BERRY BREAD WITH CHIA SEEDS

PREP TIME: 10 MINUTES ★ COOK TIME: 45 MINUTES ★ SERVINGS: 10

I've been experimenting with keto bread for a long time, and this is a winner. If you like fruity breads, you'll love this one. Enjoy a slice at breakfast with some scrambled eggs—or as a snack.

¼ cup coconut oil, melted, plus more for the pan

3 large eggs

¼ cup granulated erythritol

1 teaspoon vanilla extract

Grated zest of 1 lemon

1½ cups + 1 tablespoon almond flour

2 tablespoons psyllium husk powder

2 teaspoons baking powder

¼ teaspoon Celtic sea salt

2 tablespoons chia seeds

⅓ cup whole milk

½ cup blueberries

½ cup raspberries

1. Preheat the oven to 350°F. Grease a 9 x 5-inch loaf pan with coconut oil and line with parchment paper, going up two sides of the pan.

2. In a large bowl, whisk together the coconut oil, eggs, erythritol, vanilla, and lemon zest until smooth. In a medium bowl, combine the 1½ cups almond flour, the psyllium husk powder, baking powder, sea salt, and chia seeds. Add the almond flour mixture to the oil/egg mixture and gently fold to combine. Stir in the milk until incorporated. Set aside for 5 minutes for the chia seeds to absorb the liquid.

3. In a small bowl, combine the blueberries, raspberries, and remaining 1 tablespoon almond flour and toss to combine (the almond flour will prevent the berries from sinking in the bread). Fold the berries into the batter.

4. Scrape the batter into the prepared pan and smooth the top. Bake until an inserted toothpick comes out clean, 40 to 45 minutes. Allow to cool for 10 minutes in the pan, then remove to a wire rack to cool completely. Slice and serve.

PER SERVING ★ CALORIES: 199 ★ GRAMS OF PROTEIN: 6 ★ GRAMS OF FAT: 17 ★ GRAMS OF CARBOHYDRATE: 9 ★ PERCENT OF PROTEIN: 11% ★ PERCENT OF FAT: 72% ★ PERCENT OF CARBOHYDRATE: 17%

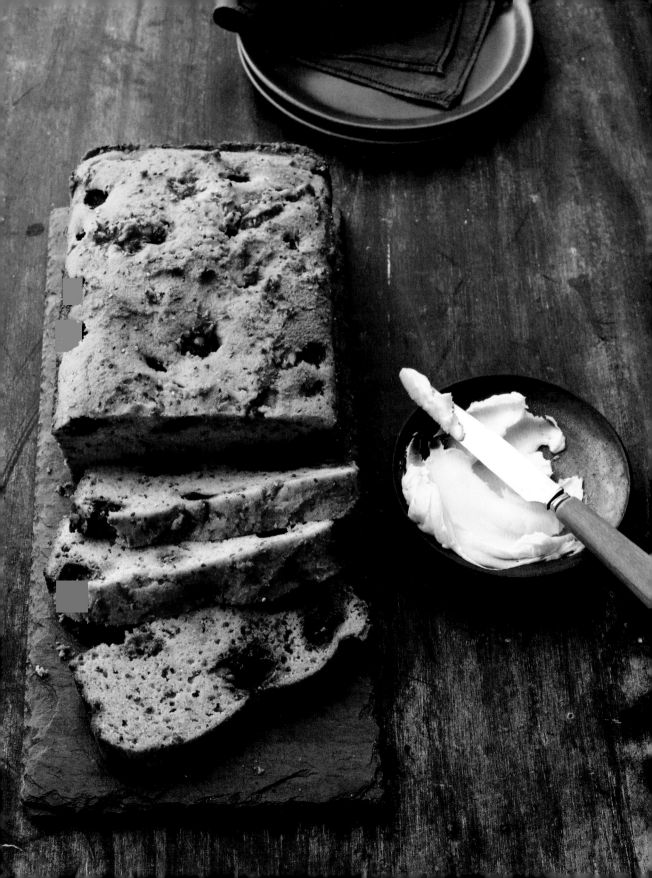

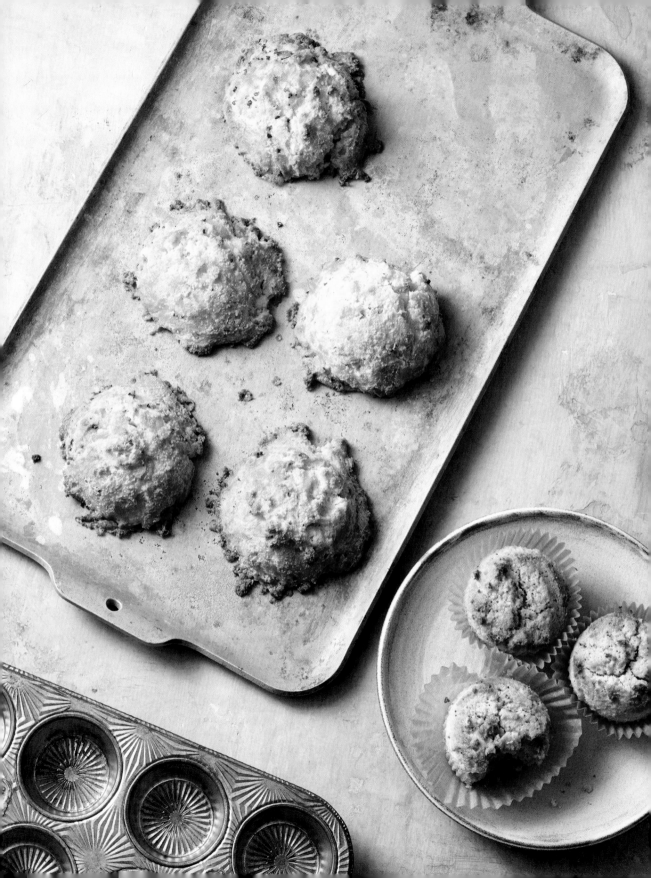

CHEDDAR AND CHIVE BISCUITS

PREP TIME: 15 MINUTES + 20 MINUTES REFRIGERATION ★ COOK TIME: 10 MINUTES ★ SERVINGS: 6

There's a chain of seafood restaurants that bakes up melt-in-your-mouth biscuits that are simply irresistible. Here's a copycat recipe that's light and loaded with buttery flavor.

1¾ cups almond flour

1 tablespoon baking powder

¼ teaspoon Celtic sea salt

¼ teaspoon freshly ground black pepper

4 tablespoons cold unsalted grass-fed butter, cubed

1 large egg, beaten

½ cup sour cream

½ cup grated sharp cheddar cheese

2 tablespoons chopped fresh chives

1. Preheat the oven to 425°F. Line a baking sheet with parchment paper.

2. In a large bowl, whisk together the almond flour, baking powder, sea salt, and pepper until combined. Add the butter and press it into the flour mixture using your fingers until pea-sized pieces form. Add the egg and sour cream and stir until just combined. Add the cheddar and chives and stir gently to incorporate. Refrigerate the mixture for 20 minutes.

3. Drop 6 biscuits (about ⅓ cup each) onto the prepared baking sheet. Bake until golden brown and puffed, 8 to 10 minutes. Allow to cool on the pan for 5 minutes before serving warm.

PER SERVING ★ CALORIES: 342 ★ GRAMS OF PROTEIN: 11 ★ GRAMS OF FAT: 32 ★ GRAMS OF CARBOHYDRATE: 9 ★ PERCENT OF PROTEIN: 12% ★ PERCENT OF FAT: 78% ★ PERCENT OF CARBOHYDRATE: 10%

LEMON POPPYSEED MUFFINS

PREP TIME: 10 MINUTES ★ COOK TIME: 18 MINUTES ★ SERVINGS: 12

Lemon poppyseed muffins are a classic comfort food. Now you can enjoy them without developing that dreaded "muffin top."

2½ cups almond flour

½ cup granulated erythritol

2 teaspoons baking powder

1 tablespoon psyllium husk powder

½ teaspoon Celtic sea salt

⅓ cup unsalted grass-fed butter, melted

½ cup heavy cream

3 large eggs, beaten

1 teaspoon vanilla extract

Grated zest of 2 medium lemons

1 tablespoon poppyseeds

Pinch of freshly grated nutmeg

1. Preheat the oven to 350°F. Line 12 cups of a muffin tin with liners.

2. In a large bowl, whisk together the almond flour, erythritol, baking powder, psyllium husk powder, and sea salt. In a medium bowl, mix together the melted butter, cream, eggs, vanilla, lemon zest, poppyseeds, and nutmeg. Pour the butter mixture into the almond flour mixture and gently fold with a rubber spatula until all of the ingredients are combined.

3. Spoon the batter evenly into the prepared muffin cups, filling each about two-thirds full. Bake until an inserted toothpick comes out clean, 15 to 18 minutes. Allow to cool in the pan for 10 minutes, then remove to a wire rack to cool completely.

PER SERVING ★ CALORIES: 109 ★ GRAMS OF PROTEIN: 2 ★ GRAMS OF FAT: 8 ★ GRAMS OF CARBOHYDRATE: 7 ★ PERCENT OF PROTEIN: 7% ★ PERCENT OF FAT: 66% ★ PERCENT OF CARBOHYDRATE: 27%

CHOCOLATE-GLAZED DOUGHNUTS

PREP TIME: 15 MINUTES ★ COOK TIME: 17 MINUTES ★ SERVINGS: 12

Think you have to give up doughnuts? Not anymore! One of these delectable pieces of goodness makes a filling breakfast, served with a piping-hot cup of coffee or espresso. As with all keto breads and pastries, it's made with low-carb almond flour.

1 cup almond flour

¼ cup granulated erythritol

1½ teaspoons baking powder

½ teaspoon Celtic sea salt

⅓ cup unsalted grass-fed butter, melted, plus more for the pan

¼ cup whole milk

3 large eggs, beaten

1 teaspoon vanilla extract

CHOCOLATE GLAZE

½ cup stevia-sweetened dark chocolate baking chips (such as Lily's)

½ cup heavy cream

2 tablespoons granulated erythritol

2 tablespoons coconut oil, melted

1. Preheat the oven to 350°F. Grease two 6-hole doughnut pans with melted butter.

2. In a large bowl, whisk together the almond flour, erythritol, baking powder, and sea salt. In a medium bowl, mix together the melted butter, milk, eggs, and vanilla until smooth. Pour the butter mixture into the almond flour mixture and stir to combine.

3. Scrape the batter into the prepared pans, filling the doughnut cavities two-thirds full. Bake until an inserted toothpick comes out clean and the doughnuts are golden brown, 12 to 15 minutes. Allow to cool in the pans for 10 minutes, then remove from the pans to a wire rack to cool completely.

4. MAKE THE CHOCOLATE GLAZE: Place the chocolate chips in a heatproof bowl. Heat the cream in the microwave or in a saucepan on the stove until warm. Pour over the chocolate chips; allow to sit for 5 minutes, then stir until smooth. Add the erythritol and coconut oil and stir until dissolved.

5. Dip the doughnuts into the chocolate glaze and place back on the wire rack. Allow the glaze to set before serving.

PER SERVING ★ CALORIES: 241 ★ GRAMS OF PROTEIN: 4 ★ GRAMS OF FAT: 21 ★ GRAMS OF CARBOHYDRATE: 9 ★ PERCENT OF PROTEIN: 7% ★ PERCENT OF FAT: 78% ★ PERCENT OF CARBOHYDRATE: 15%

CINNAMON ROLL BITES

PREP TIME: 15 MINUTES + 30 MINUTES REFRIGERATION ★ COOK TIME: 20 MINUTES
★ SERVINGS: 16

I've cloned one of the world's best cinnamon rolls with this recipe. Start baking these, and that magical cinnamon aroma will waft through your house and draw everyone to the kitchen. These rolls are the ultimate comfort food at breakfast.

CINNAMON ROLL DOUGH

1 (8-ounce) container full-fat cream cheese, at room temperature

2½ cups shredded low-moisture whole-milk mozzarella cheese

¾ cup almond flour

⅓ cup coconut flour

⅓ cup granulated erythritol

2 tablespoons baking powder

1 teaspoon vanilla extract

¼ teaspoon Celtic sea salt

3 large eggs, beaten

2 tablespoons unsalted grass-fed butter, melted

1. PREPARE THE CINNAMON ROLL DOUGH: In a large microwave-safe bowl, combine the cream cheese and mozzarella and heat in the microwave in 30-second intervals, stirring after each, until melted and smooth. Add the almond flour, coconut flour, erythritol, baking powder, vanilla, sea salt, and eggs and stir until combined and a dough forms. Cover and refrigerate for 30 minutes.

2. Preheat the oven to 400°F. Grease an 8 x 8-inch baking pan with the 2 tablespoons melted butter.

3. MAKE THE CINNAMON ROLLS: Roll the dough out between two pieces of parchment paper to a 15 x 10-inch rectangle ¼ inch thick. Brush the melted butter over the dough. In a small bowl, combine the erythritol and cinnamon. Evenly sprinkle the cinnamon mixture over the dough. Starting at the long side, roll the dough up in a jelly-roll fashion. Cut crosswise into 8 wheels. Then cut each wheel in half to make 16 bites.

4. Arrange in the baking dish, spiral-side up, and bake until golden, 18 to 20 minutes. Allow to cool almost completely before frosting.

PER SERVING ★ CALORIES: 258 ★ GRAMS OF PROTEIN: 8 ★ GRAMS OF FAT: 22 ★ GRAMS OF CARBOHYDRATE: 5 ★ PERCENT OF PROTEIN: 13% ★ PERCENT OF FAT: 78% ★ PERCENT OF CARBOHYDRATE: 9%

CINNAMON ROLL FILLING

2 tablespoons unsalted grass-fed butter, melted

⅓ cup granulated erythritol

2 tablespoons ground cinnamon

CINNAMON ROLL FROSTING

4 ounces full-fat cream cheese, at room temperature

¼ cup granulated erythritol

2 tablespoons heavy cream

½ teaspoon vanilla extract

5. MEANWHILE, MAKE THE CINNAMON ROLL FROSTING: In a bowl, mix together the cream cheese, erythritol, cream, and vanilla until smooth.

6. Just before serving, spread the frosting on top of the rolls.

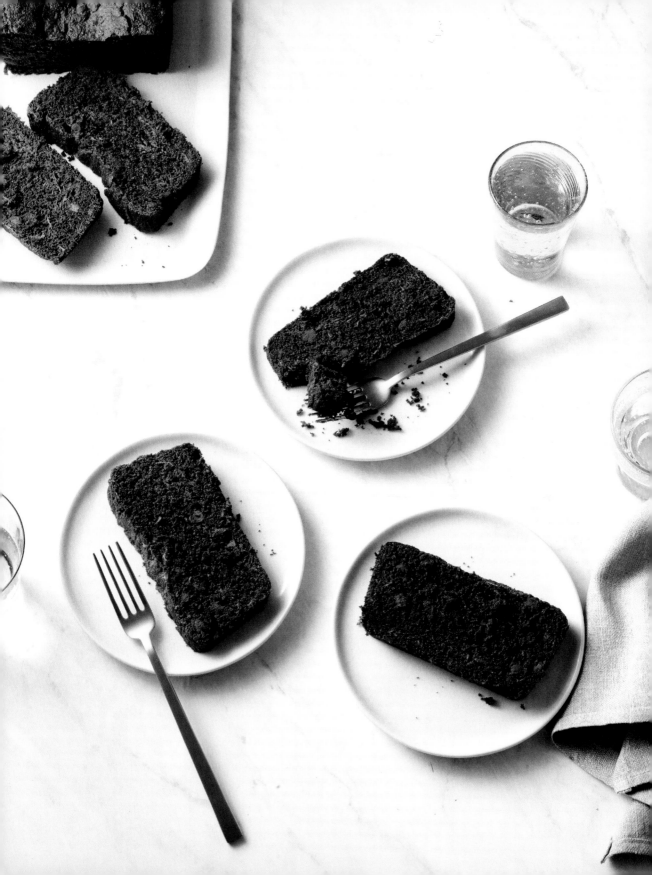

CHOCOLATE ZUCCHINI BREAD

PREP TIME: 10 MINUTES ★ COOK TIME: 1 HOUR ★ SERVINGS: 8

I'm crazy about zucchini bread, but I don't like all the sugar traditional versions contain. So I've sweetened it up with chocolate chips (for a chocolaty twist) and erythritol. There's lots of yummy zucchini in the mix, too—for extra fiber and nutrients.

½ cup unsweetened cocoa powder

½ teaspoon Celtic sea salt

1½ cups almond flour

1 teaspoon baking soda

1½ teaspoons baking powder

8 tablespoons (1 stick) unsalted grass-fed butter, at room temperature, plus melted butter for the pan

⅔ cup granulated erythritol

3 large eggs

1 teaspoon vanilla extract

1½ cups grated zucchini, squeezed of excess liquid

½ cup stevia-sweetened dark chocolate baking chips (such as Lily's)

1. Preheat the oven to 350°F. Grease a 9 x 5-inch loaf pan with melted butter. Line it with parchment paper, going up two sides of the pan, and grease the parchment with additional melted butter.

2. In a large bowl, whisk together the cocoa powder, sea salt, almond flour, baking soda, and baking powder.

3. In a bowl with a hand mixer (or in a stand mixer fitted with the paddle attachment), beat the butter and erythritol until combined and fluffy. Add the eggs one at a time, mixing until just incorporated. Beat in the vanilla. Add the cocoa powder mixture to the butter/egg mixture and mix until just combined. Gently fold in the zucchini and chocolate chips using a rubber spatula.

4. Scrape the batter into the prepared pan. Bake until an inserted toothpick comes out clean, 45 minutes to 1 hour. Allow to cool in the pan for 10 minutes, then remove to a wire rack to cool completely.

5. Store in the refrigerator to keep moist.

PER SERVING ★ CALORIES: 353 ★ GRAMS OF PROTEIN: 9 ★ GRAMS OF FAT: 29 ★ GRAMS OF CARBOHYDRATE: 14 ★ PERCENT OF PROTEIN: 10% ★ PERCENT OF FAT: 74% ★ PERCENT OF CARBOHYDRATE: 16%

KETO DINNER ROLLS

PREP TIME: 5 MINUTES + 20 MINUTES REFRIGERATION ★ COOK TIME: 25 MINUTES ★ SERVINGS: 8

No longer do you have to wave off the bread basket, thanks to these amazing dinner rolls. If you've missed bread at your evening meals, welcome it back with open arms—and an open mouth!

1½ cups shredded low-moisture whole-milk mozzarella cheese

4 ounces full-fat cream cheese

1½ cups superfine almond flour

1 tablespoon baking powder

½ teaspoon Celtic sea salt

3 large eggs

2 tablespoons unsalted grass-fed butter, melted, plus more for greasing

1. Preheat the oven to 375°F. Line a baking sheet with parchment paper.

2. In a large microwave-safe bowl, combine the mozzarella and cream cheese and heat in the microwave in 15-second intervals, stirring after each, until melted and smooth. Add the almond flour, baking powder, sea salt, and eggs and mix until combined into a dough (using your hands is best until everything is incorporated). Refrigerate the dough for 20 minutes.

3. Grease your hands with a little butter and form the dough into 8 smooth balls. Place on the prepared baking sheet about 1 inch apart.

4. Brush the rolls with 1 tablespoon of the melted butter. Bake until puffed and golden, 20 to 25 minutes. Remove from the oven and brush with the remaining 1 tablespoon melted butter. Serve warm.

PER SERVING ★ CALORIES: 222 ★ GRAMS OF PROTEIN: 11 ★ GRAMS OF FAT: 17 ★ GRAMS OF CARBOHYDRATE: 5 ★ PERCENT OF PROTEIN: 21% ★ PERCENT OF FAT: 69% ★ PERCENT OF CARBOHYDRATE: 10%

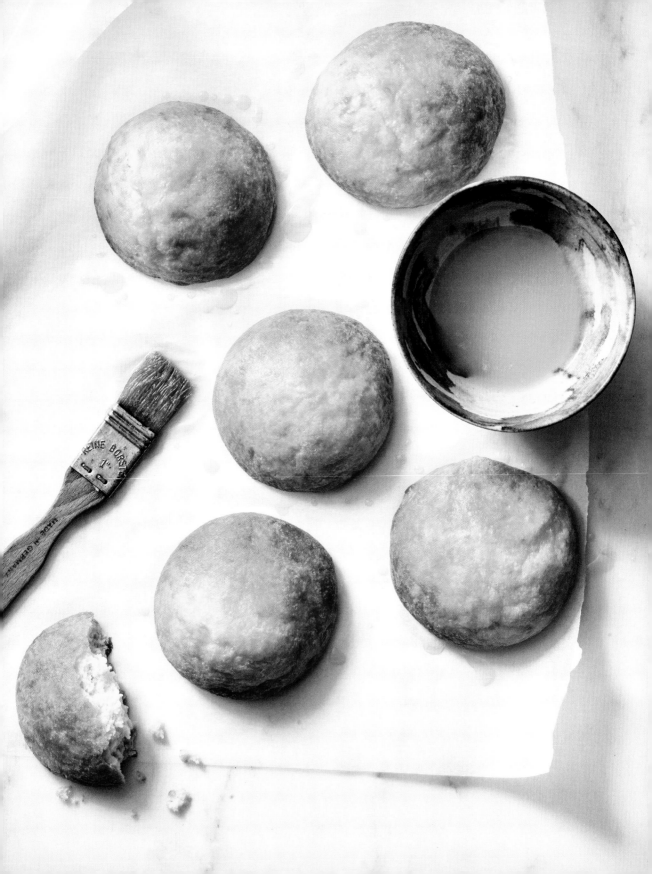

BREAKFASTS

Each morning, if you're not doing intermittent fasting, choose one of these breakfasts. Have a different breakfast every day, or stick to a few breakfasts you love.

These recipes remove the excess carbs that put you on a roller coaster of insulin and blood-sugar spikes and restrict your body's ability to burn fat. This helps your body tap into fat stores for energy, resulting in the loss of inches and fat.

Get ready to enjoy keto-friendly pancakes, waffles, bacon, and more in the morning!

SOUTHWESTERN FRITTATA WITH CHORIZO

PREP TIME: 8 MINUTES ★ COOK TIME: 23 MINUTES ★ SERVES: 8

A frittata is a traditional Italian dish (I was practically weaned on them) with eggs, vegetables, and herbs. This frittata is made with peppers, onions, cheese, and chorizo, a type of pork sausage. Starting your morning with a frittata will keep you satisfied all day long.

4 large eggs

2 egg yolks, beaten

2 tablespoons extra-virgin olive oil

6 ounces fresh chorizo, casings removed

½ red bell pepper, finely diced

½ yellow onion, diced

2 cloves garlic, minced

1½ teaspoons ground cumin

2 teaspoons chili powder

Celtic sea salt

Freshly ground black pepper

½ cup shredded sharp cheddar cheese

Chopped fresh cilantro, for garnish

1. Preheat the oven to 400°F.

2. In a bowl, beat together the whole eggs and egg yolks and set aside.

3. In a 10-inch nonstick ovenproof or cast-iron skillet, heat the olive oil over medium-high heat. Add the chorizo and, without stirring, allow to brown, about 4 minutes. Break up the chorizo using the back of a wooden spoon and allow to brown another 4 minutes. Using a slotted spoon, remove the chorizo to a plate lined with paper towels.

4. Add the bell pepper and onion to the pan and cook until softened, 5 to 6 minutes. Add the garlic, cumin, and chili powder during the last minute. Season to taste with salt and pepper. Sprinkle the chorizo and cheddar into the pan. Add the beaten eggs and allow the edges to set, about 2 minutes.

5. Transfer the skillet to the oven and bake until the eggs are just set in the center, 6 to 7 minutes. Allow to cool for 5 minutes before serving garnished with cilantro.

PER SERVING ★ CALORIES: 210 ★ GRAMS OF PROTEIN: 11 ★ GRAMS OF FAT: 17 ★ GRAMS OF CARBOHYDRATE: 3 ★ PERCENT OF PROTEIN: 21% ★ PERCENT OF FAT: 73% ★ PERCENT OF CARBOHYDRATE: 6%

BLUEBERRY PANCAKES

PREP TIME: 10 MINUTES ★ COOK TIME: 15 MINUTES ★ SERVINGS: 4

A couple of blueberry pancakes at a typical pancake restaurant serves up 60 grams of carbs or more—way too much for keto dieters and their waistlines. I've got a better version that delivers the same flavor with a fraction of the carbs. This recipe weighs in at only 20 grams—quite a savings.

PANCAKES

6 ounces full-fat cream cheese, at room temperature

4 large eggs, beaten

2 teaspoons vanilla extract

⅔ cup coconut flour

2 teaspoons baking powder

¼ cup granulated erythritol

½ teaspoon ground cinnamon

2 teaspoons grated lemon zest

¼ cup blueberries

4 tablespoons unsalted grass-fed butter, for the pan

SAUCE

¼ cup blueberries

1 tablespoon granulated erythritol

1 tablespoon water

1 tablespoon fresh lemon juice

1. MAKE THE PANCAKES: In a bowl, mix together the cream cheese, eggs, and vanilla until smooth. In a separate bowl, combine the coconut flour, baking powder, erythritol, and cinnamon. Add the flour mixture to the cream cheese mixture and stir to combine. Gently fold in the lemon zest and blueberries.

2. Heat a large nonstick skillet or griddle over medium-high heat and add 2 teaspoons of the butter. Use a ¼-cup measure to scoop pancake batter into the pan—for 2 to 3 pancakes. Allow to cook until golden brown on one side and small bubbles form, 3 to 4 minutes. Flip and allow to cook on the other side until golden brown and cooked through, another 2 minutes. Repeat with the remaining batter, buttering the pan if necessary.

3. MAKE THE SAUCE: In a food processor, pulse together the blueberries, erythritol, water, and lemon juice until smooth. Drizzle 1 tablespoon over each serving.

PER SERVING ★ CALORIES: 418 ★ GRAMS OF PROTEIN: 12 ★ GRAMS OF FAT: 33 ★ GRAMS OF CARBOHYDRATE: 20 ★ PERCENT OF PROTEIN: 11% ★ PERCENT OF FAT: 70% ★ PERCENT OF CARBOHYDRATE: 19%

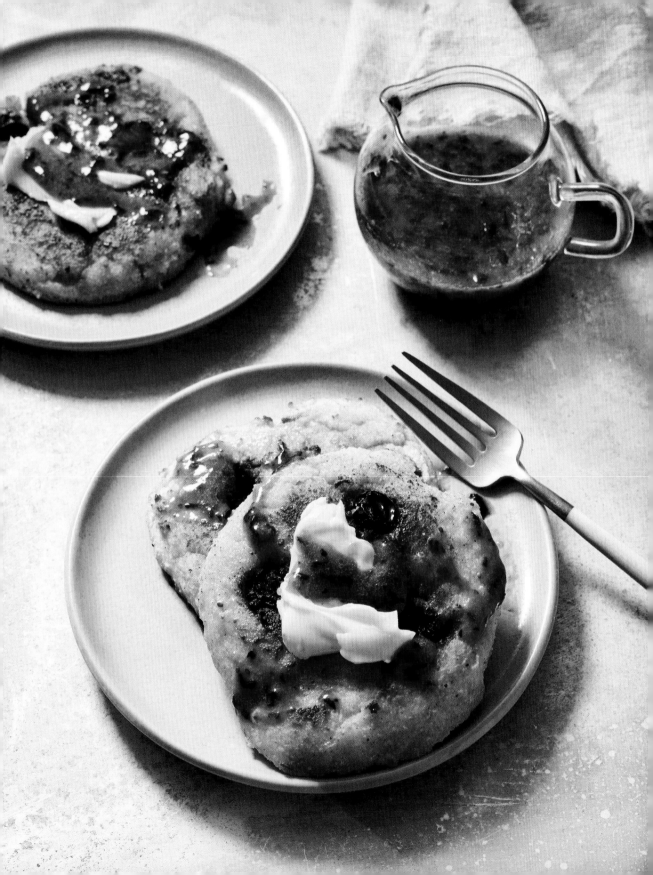

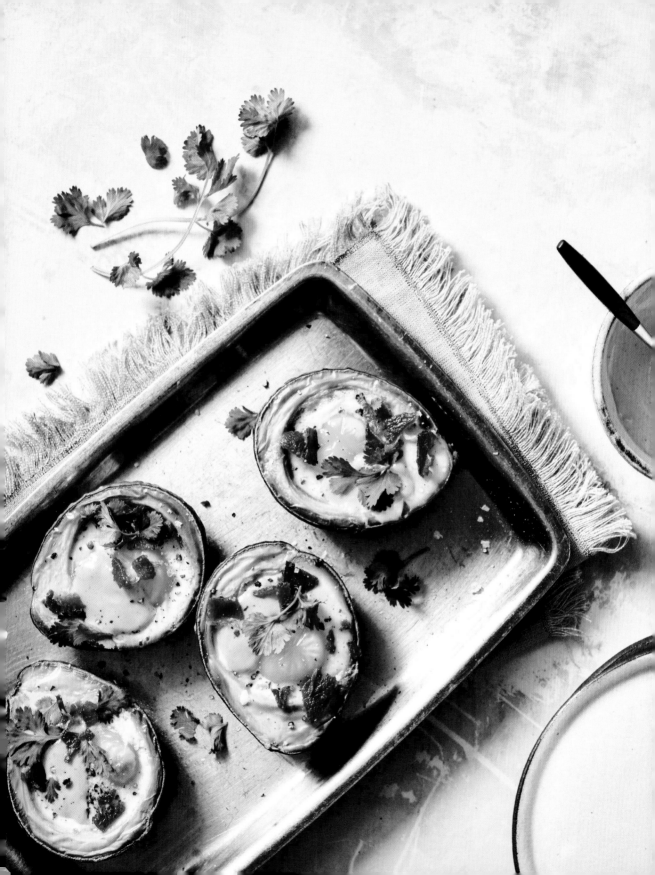

EGG IN AN AVOCADO WITH BACON

PREP TIME: 10 MINUTES ★ COOK TIME: 20 MINUTES, INCLUDING 5 MINUTES TO PAN-FRY THE BACON ★ SERVINGS: 4

Calling all avocado lovers: here's a simple and tasty recipe that pairs two of the most delicious fats on the planet (bacon and avocado) with a serving of hearty eggs.

2 large avocados, halved and pitted

4 large eggs

Celtic sea salt and freshly ground black pepper

⅓ cup mayonnaise (store-bought, preferably olive oil–based)

1 clove garlic, grated

2 tablespoons Sriracha

4 slices bacon, cooked and crumbled

Chopped fresh cilantro, for garnish

1. Preheat the oven to 425°F.

2. Scoop a little flesh out of the avocado halves and place them on a baking sheet. Place an egg in the hole of each avocado half and season to taste with salt and pepper. Bake until the whites are set and the yolks are still runny, 12 to 15 minutes.

3. Meanwhile, in a small bowl, combine the mayonnaise, garlic, and Sriracha. Set aside until ready to serve.

4. When the avocados are done, serve topped with the crumbled bacon, cilantro, and a dollop of the spicy mayo.

PER SERVING ★ CALORIES: 351 ★ GRAMS OF PROTEIN: 6 ★ GRAMS OF FAT: 32 ★ GRAMS OF CARBOHYDRATE: 11 ★ PERCENT OF PROTEIN: 11% ★ PERCENT OF FAT: 79% ★ PERCENT OF CARBOHYDRATE: 10%

ITALIAN-SPICED EGGS IN TOMATO SAUCE WITH RICOTTA

PREP TIME: 10 MINUTES ★ COOK TIME: 16 MINUTES ★ SERVINGS: 4

When Italian families like mine get together for reunions, a big breakfast begins the celebration. It's something like this dish—cooked eggs buried under a blanket of rich, spiced-right tomato sauce. This recipe works well for brunch, too.

2 tablespoons extra-virgin olive oil

½ yellow onion, finely diced

2 cloves garlic, minced

1½ teaspoons dried oregano

1 teaspoon dried thyme

⅛ teaspoon red pepper flakes

Celtic sea salt

Freshly ground black pepper

2 cups baby spinach

2 cups crushed canned tomatoes

4 large eggs

1 cup whole-milk ricotta cheese

2 tablespoons chopped fresh parsley, for garnish

1. Position the oven rack so that it is 5 inches from the broiler, and preheat the oven to broil.

2. In a cast-iron skillet or heavy-bottomed ovenproof pan, heat the olive oil over medium-high heat. Add the onion and cook until softened, about 5 minutes. Add the garlic, oregano, thyme, pepper flakes, and salt and black pepper to taste. Add the spinach and allow to wilt. Add the crushed tomatoes, season again with salt and black pepper, and bring to a simmer.

3. Make 4 small nests for the eggs and drop the eggs into the sauce. Season the eggs with salt and pepper. Dollop the ricotta around the tomato sauce. Place under the broiler and broil until the egg whites are set but the yolks are still runny, 5 to 8 minutes.

4. Serve hot, garnished with the parsley.

PER SERVING ★ CALORIES: 294 ★ GRAMS OF PROTEIN: 16 ★ GRAMS OF FAT: 20 ★ GRAMS OF CARBOHYDRATE: 14 ★ PERCENT OF PROTEIN: 22% ★ PERCENT OF FAT: 60% ★ PERCENT OF CARBOHYDRATE: 18%

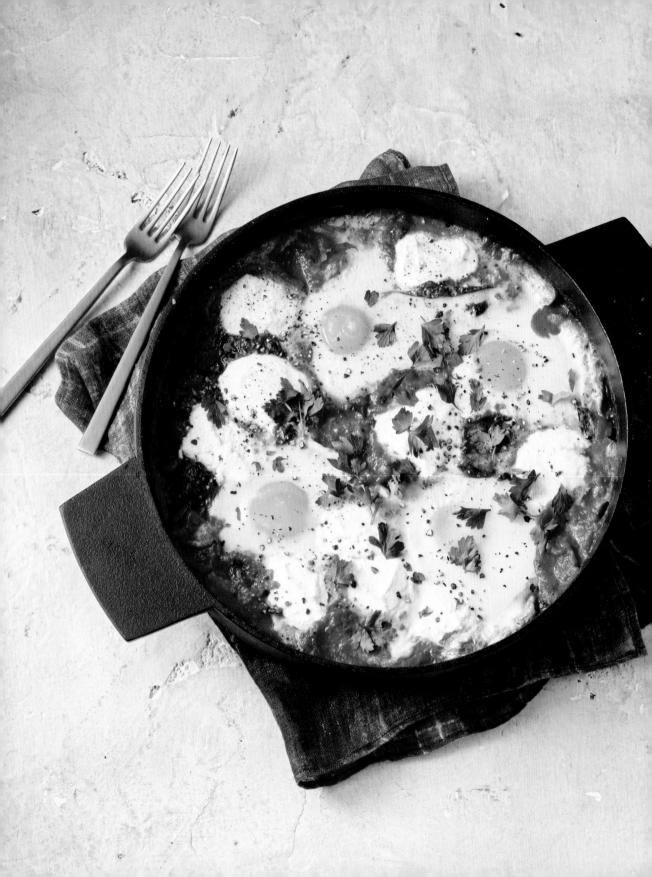

GRAIN-FREE GRANOLA

PREP TIME: 10 MINUTES ★ COOK TIME: 30 MINUTES ★ MAKES: 3½ CUPS (¼ CUP PER SERVING)
★ SERVINGS: 14

Store-bought granola masquerades as a health food, but it's often
loaded with sugar, questionable fats, and preservatives. Here's my
rendition of granola but without the sugar and carbs that plague
most granolas. Rather than oats, to cut carbs I've used nuts and
seeds. You won't be able to tell the difference between this granola
and its carb-filled counterparts. This granola tastes yummy with
Greek yogurt or a nut milk.

1 cup unsweetened coconut
flakes

1 cup sliced almonds

½ cup pecan halves, roughly
chopped

½ cup sunflower seeds

½ cup hulled pumpkin seeds
(pepitas)

2 tablespoons sesame seeds

½ teaspoon Celtic sea salt

¾ teaspoon ground cinnamon

¼ cup granulated erythritol

1 teaspoon vanilla extract

¼ cup coconut oil, melted

1. Preheat the oven to 300°F. Line two baking sheets with
parchment paper.

2. In a large bowl, combine all of the ingredients and mix
to evenly coat. Spread out on the prepared baking sheets
and bake until golden brown, 25 to 30 minutes, stirring
halfway through. Remove and allow to cool. Break into
pieces. The granola can be stored in a sealed container in
your pantry or refrigerator.

PER SERVING ★ CALORIES: 232 ★ GRAMS OF PROTEIN: 5 ★ GRAMS OF FAT: 21 ★ GRAMS OF CARBOHYDRATE: 7 ★
PERCENT OF PROTEIN: 8% ★ PERCENT OF FAT: 84% ★ PERCENT OF CARBOHYDRATE: 8%

FRIED EGGS IN BROWNED BUTTER WITH ASPARAGUS AND HOLLANDAISE

PREP TIME: 5 MINUTES ★ COOK TIME: 20 MINUTES ★ SERVINGS: 4

If you savor sinking a fork into a perfectly cooked egg bathed in hollandaise sauce, you'll appreciate this keto version of Eggs Benedict. It subs out the usual starchy muffin for asparagus—which I find tastier and infinitely healthier.

HOLLANDAISE

3 egg yolks

1 teaspoon fresh lemon juice

Pinch of cayenne pepper

6 tablespoons ghee, melted

Celtic sea salt

Pinch of ground white pepper

EGGS AND ASPARAGUS

1 small bunch asparagus, ends trimmed

2 tablespoons unsalted grass-fed butter

4 large eggs

Celtic sea salt

Freshly ground black pepper

2 tablespoons sliced fresh chives, for garnish

1. MAKE THE HOLLANDAISE: In a blender, combine the egg yolks, lemon juice, and cayenne and blend until smooth. With the machine running, slowly stream in the melted ghee until a sauce forms and is emulsified. Season with sea salt to taste and the white pepper. If the sauce is too thick, add a little bit of warm water and pulse again to combine.

2. PREPARE THE EGGS AND ASPARAGUS: Set up a large bowl of ice and water and set it near the stove. Bring a medium saucepan of water to a boil.

3. Add the asparagus to the boiling water and cook until bright green and almost tender, about 5 minutes. Transfer to the ice bath to cool. (Hold on to the pan of hot water.) Drain the asparagus and pat dry with paper towels.

4. In a nonstick sauté pan, heat the butter over medium heat. When the butter begins to foam and turn light brown and nutty, add the eggs and season to taste with salt and black pepper. Allow the eggs to cook until the whites are set but the yolks are still runny, about 5 minutes.

(recipe continues)

5. Reheat the asparagus in hot water for a couple of seconds. Dry on paper towels and place a few stalks on each plate. Top with a fried egg and browned butter. Drizzle with hollandaise sauce and garnish with chives.

PER SERVING ★ CALORIES: 362 ★ GRAMS OF PROTEIN: 10 ★ GRAMS OF FAT: 35 ★ GRAMS OF CARBOHYDRATE: 4 ★ PERCENT OF PROTEIN: 11% ★ PERCENT OF FAT: 85% ★ PERCENT OF CARBOHYDRATE: 4%

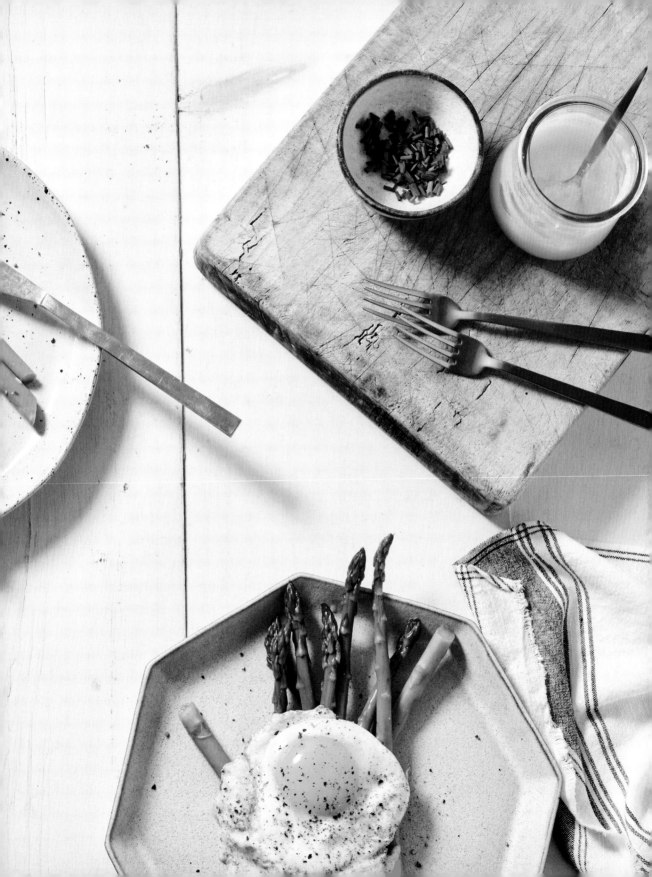

CHOCOLATE CHIP WAFFLES

PREP TIME: 10 MINUTES ★ COOK TIME: 15 MINUTES ★ SERVINGS: 8

I love waffles. Bring them on! But don't bring them with a lot of carbs. My love affair with this usually decadent breakfast dish motivated me to create a keto version, complete with chocolate chips. Now I can have my waffles and eat them, too.

6 tablespoons unsalted grass-fed butter

½ cup nut butter of your choice (I use creamy unsweetened natural peanut butter)

4 large egg yolks

1½ teaspoons vanilla extract

2 cups almond flour

3 tablespoons granulated erythritol

1½ teaspoons baking powder

1 teaspoon Celtic sea salt

¾ cup whole milk

½ cup stevia-sweetened dark chocolate baking chips (such as Lily's)

Olive oil or avocado oil cooking spray

1. In a small microwave-safe bowl, combine the butter and nut butter and heat in 15-second intervals, stirring after each, until melted and smooth. Place the egg yolks in another small bowl. Whisk the nut butter mixture into the egg yolks and add the vanilla.

2. In a large bowl, combine the almond flour, erythritol, baking powder, and sea salt and mix well. Pour the egg yolk mixture into the almond flour mixture and mix to combine. Stir in the milk until the batter is smooth, then fold in the chocolate chips.

3. Preheat a waffle iron. Coat the waffle iron with cooking spray.

4. Pour ⅓ cup of the waffle batter into the waffle iron (or more depending on the size of your waffle iron) and close. Cook according to the manufacturer's instructions. Remove the waffle and continue with the remaining batter.

PER SERVING ★ CALORIES: 369 ★ GRAMS OF PROTEIN: 13 ★ GRAMS OF FAT: 32 ★ GRAMS OF CARBOHYDRATE: 11 ★ PERCENT OF PROTEIN: 11% ★ PERCENT OF FAT: 74% ★ PERCENT OF CARBOHYDRATE: 15%

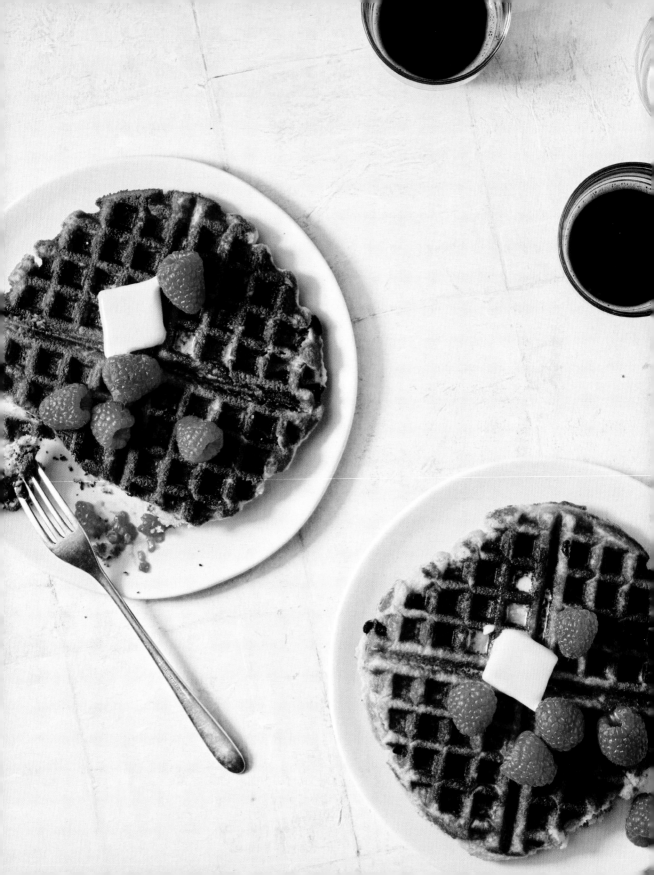

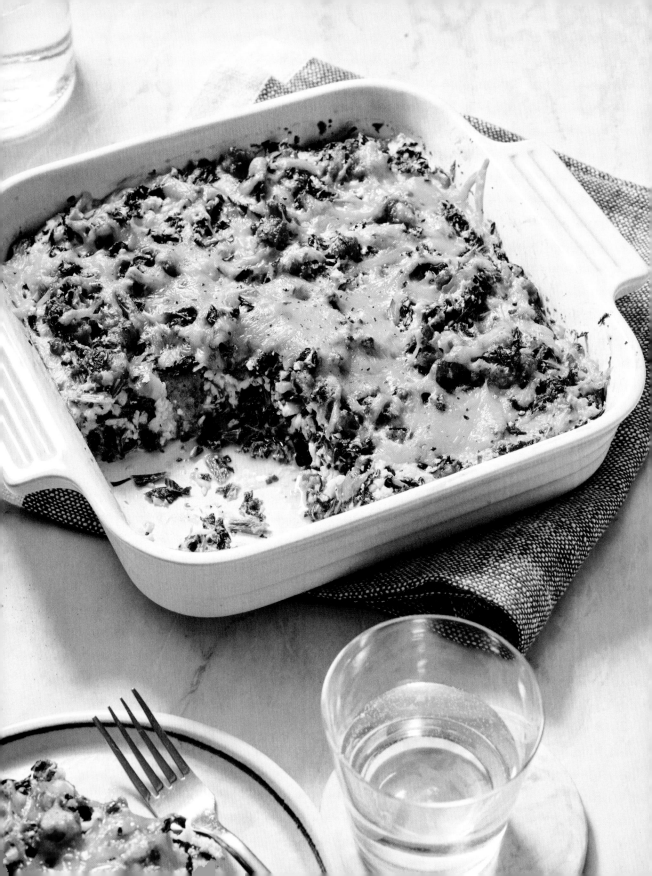

"HASH BROWN" BREAKFAST BAKE

PREP TIME: 20 MINUTES ★ COOK TIME: 40 MINUTES ★ SERVINGS: 6

Now-trendy cauliflower is a stand-in for hash browns here. And what a stand-in it is! Properly prepared "riced" cauliflower delivers four times fewer calories and more fiber than potatoes. It ranks high on my list of keto foods.

Olive oil or avocado oil cooking spray

2 cups small cauliflower florets

1 tablespoon extra-virgin olive oil

8 ounces fresh sugar-free breakfast sausage, casings removed

6 large eggs

½ cup heavy cream

1 (10-ounce) package frozen spinach, thawed and squeezed of excess liquid

Celtic sea salt

Freshly ground black pepper

1½ cups shredded sharp cheddar cheese

1. Preheat the oven to 350°F. Coat an 8 x 8-inch baking dish with cooking spray.

2. In a food processor, pulse the cauliflower florets until they resemble rice. Set aside.

3. In a sauté pan, heat the olive oil over medium-high heat. Add the sausage and allow to brown, about 5 minutes. Break the sausage up with the back of a wooden spoon and continue to brown it, another 5 minutes. Remove the sausage to a plate lined with paper towels and allow to cool.

4. In a medium bowl, whisk together the eggs and cream until combined. Add the spinach and season with salt and pepper. Add ¾ cup of the cheddar and mix.

5. Pour the egg/spinach/cheese mixture into the baking dish and add the cooked sausage and cauliflower rice. Sprinkle the top with the remaining cheddar.

6. Bake until golden and puffed and a toothpick inserted in the center comes out clean, 25 to 30 minutes.

PER SERVING ★ CALORIES: 331 ★ GRAMS OF PROTEIN: 22 ★ GRAMS OF FAT: 24 ★ GRAMS OF CARBOHYDRATE: 6 ★ PERCENT OF PROTEIN: 27% ★ PERCENT OF FAT: 65% ★ PERCENT OF CARBOHYDRATE: 8%

APPETIZERS + SNACKS

With keto breakfasts, lunches, and dinners on this diet, you still have room to snack. Try to incorporate one snack in your meal planning each day. The snacks in this chapter are made with natural ingredients, nothing overly processed, and very few carbs.

Other healthy snacks include raw veggies, cheeses, smoothies, hard-boiled eggs, Greek yogurt, and nuts and seeds.

If you love to entertain and feed a crowd, or have volunteered to bring an appetizer to a party, make it easy on your waistline. Most of these recipes are party-friendly, and guests won't even know they are keto-friendly (unless you tell them) because they taste so delicious.

AVOCADO HUMMUS

PREP TIME: 5 MINUTES ★ MAKES: 1 CUP (¼ CUP PER SERVING) ★ SERVINGS: 4

Here's a new twist on hummus—with avocado! Talk about a tasty nutritional bargain. This luscious fruit is full of healthy fats, fiber, potassium, beta-carotene, folate, and vitamin C, making it one of the best and most versatile keto foods you can eat.

1 avocado, halved and pitted

¼ cup tahini

3 tablespoons fresh lime juice

½ teaspoon Celtic sea salt

¼ teaspoon freshly ground black pepper

¼ to ½ cup hot water (optional)

2 tablespoons chopped fresh cilantro, for garnish

4 stalks celery, each cut into thirds, for serving

1. Scoop the avocado into a food processor and add the tahini, lime juice, sea salt, and pepper and pulse until smooth. If not smooth enough, add ¼ to ½ cup hot water to the food processor. (If not serving right away, refrigerate, but sprinkle with some lemon juice to keep the hummus from turning brown.)

2. Serve garnished with the cilantro, and with the celery sticks for dipping.

PER SERVING ★ CALORIES: 191 ★ GRAMS OF PROTEIN: 4 ★ GRAMS OF FAT: 15 ★ GRAMS OF CARBOHYDRATE: 10 ★ PERCENT OF PROTEIN: 8% ★ PERCENT OF FAT: 71% ★ PERCENT OF CARBOHYDRATE: 21%

CAULIFLOWER HUMMUS

PREP TIME: 5 MINUTES ★ COOK TIME: 1 HOUR 12 MINUTES, INCLUDING 1 HOUR TO ROAST GARLIC ★ MAKES: 2¼ CUPS (¼ CUP PER SERVING) ★ SERVINGS: 9

One of my favorite snacks is hummus—it's always in my fridge! But not the usual chickpea hummus. I make hummus with low-carb veggies like cauliflower, accented by all the usual hummus ingredients: garlic, tahini, and lemon juice. For keto comfort food dieters, this easy-to-make recipe is a nutritional slam dunk.

1 head cauliflower, cut into florets (about 4 cups)

¼ cup tahini

⅓ cup mayonnaise

4 cloves Roasted Garlic (recipe follows), peeled

3 tablespoons fresh lemon juice

¼ teaspoon Celtic sea salt

⅛ teaspoon ground white pepper

⅛ teaspoon smoked paprika

1 tablespoon fresh parsley, chopped

9 stalks celery, each cut into thirds, for serving

1. Bring a large pot of salted water to a boil. Add the cauliflower florets and boil until tender, 10 to 12 minutes. Drain the florets, reserving ½ cup salted cooking water.

2. Place the florets in a food processor and pulse, adding the reserved cooking water ¼ cup at a time until smooth. Add the tahini, mayonnaise, roasted garlic, lemon juice, sea salt, and white pepper.

3. Transfer to a bowl and sprinkle with the smoked paprika and chopped parsley to finish. Serve with the celery sticks.

PER SERVING ★ CALORIES: 255 ★ GRAMS OF PROTEIN: 5 ★ GRAMS OF FAT: 21 ★ GRAMS OF CARBOHYDRATE: 12 ★ PERCENT OF PROTEIN: 7% ★ PERCENT OF FAT: 75% ★ PERCENT OF CARBOHYDRATE: 18%

ROASTED GARLIC

1 bulb garlic, top cut off

1 tablespoon extra-virgin olive oil

1. Preheat the oven to 400°F.

2. Place the bulb of garlic on a piece of foil. Drizzle the garlic with the olive oil and enclose in the foil. Roast for 45 minutes to 1 hour, or until the garlic is softened and light brown. Remove and allow to cool for 10 minutes before using. You may store the leftovers in a zip-top bag or container in the refrigerator for up to 1 week.

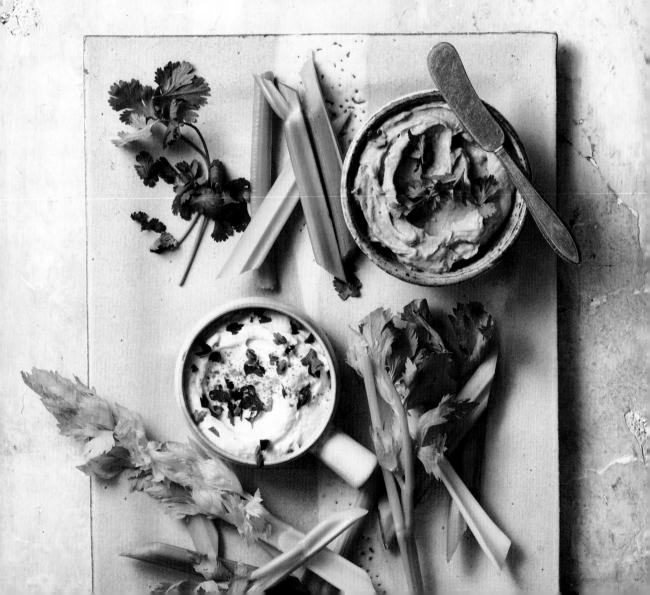

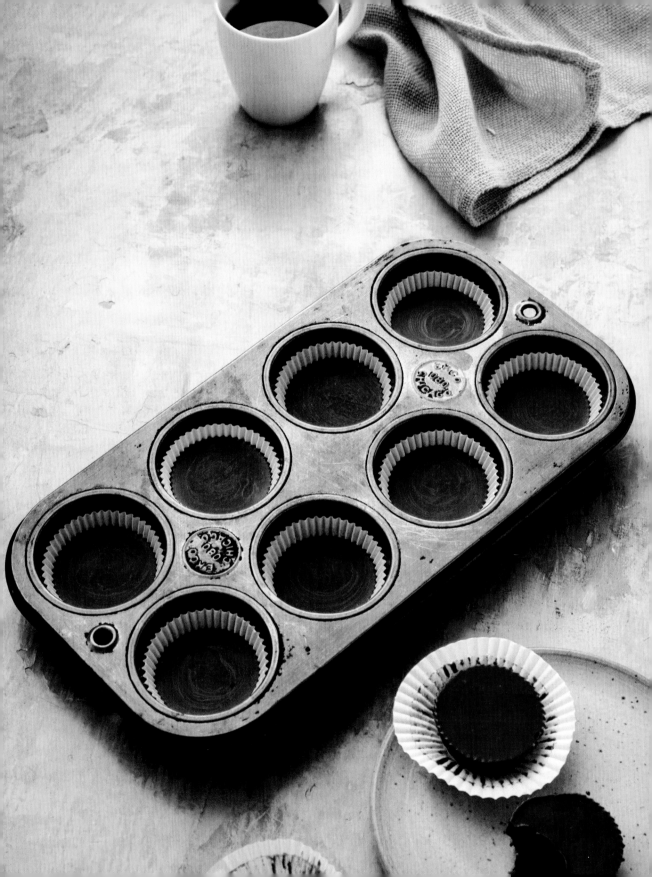

CHOCOLATE PEANUT BUTTER FAT BOMBS

PREP TIME: 5 MINUTES ★ COOK TIME: 45 MINUTES ★ SERVINGS: 16

I've said it many times: Peanut butter and chocolate is a sweet marriage made in heaven, or rather in the kitchen. These melt-in-your-mouth bombs are sugar-free and packed with keto-friendly fats. They'll detonate a flavor explosion in your mouth.

⅔ cup creamy unsweetened natural peanut butter

⅓ cup coconut oil, melted

2 tablespoons MCT oil

1 teaspoon vanilla extract

3 tablespoons confectioners' erythritol

3 tablespoons unsweetened cocoa powder

¼ teaspoon Celtic sea salt

1. Line 16 cups of a mini muffin tin with liners.

2. In a food processor, combine all the ingredients and puree until smooth. Divide the mixture evenly among the cups. Freeze until set, 30 to 45 minutes. Store in the freezer, covered, for up to 1 month.

PER SERVING ★ CALORIES: 122 ★ GRAMS OF PROTEIN: 3 ★ GRAMS OF FAT: 12 ★ GRAMS OF CARBOHYDRATE: 3 ★ PERCENT OF PROTEIN: 9% ★ PERCENT OF FAT: 82% ★ PERCENT OF CARBOHYDRATE: 9%

JALAPEÑO POPPERS WITH BACON

PREP TIME: 10 MINUTES ★ COOK TIME: 20 MINUTES ★ SERVINGS: 4

I've been known to devour this popular restaurant appetizer by the plateful. Biting into cheesy poppers and having the jalapeño heat explode in my mouth is an experience all its own. Usually these snacks are coated with a carby crust, then deep-fried. But I've wrapped them in bacon instead, and baked them to perfection. Only 3 grams of carbs will pass your lips with these treats.

4½ ounces full-fat cream cheese, at room temperature

⅓ cup shredded cheddar cheese

¼ teaspoon chili powder

1 scallion, finely chopped

⅛ teaspoon freshly ground black pepper

6 jalapeños, halved lengthwise and seeded

6 slices bacon, halved

1. Preheat the oven to 400°F. Place a wire rack inside a sheet pan.

2. In a medium bowl, blend together the cream cheese, cheddar, chili powder, scallion, and black pepper and mix to combine. Spread the cream cheese mixture evenly in the boat of the halved jalapeños. Wrap each jalapeño in a piece of bacon.

3. Place the wrapped jalapeños on the wire rack. Bake until the bacon is browned and crisp and the cheese has melted, 15 to 20 minutes. Allow to cool for 5 minutes before serving.

PER SERVING ★ CALORIES: 193 ★ GRAMS OF PROTEIN: 7 ★ GRAMS OF FAT: 17 ★ GRAMS OF CARBOHYDRATE: 3 ★ PERCENT OF PROTEIN: 15% ★ PERCENT OF FAT: 79% ★ PERCENT OF CARBOHYDRATE: 6%

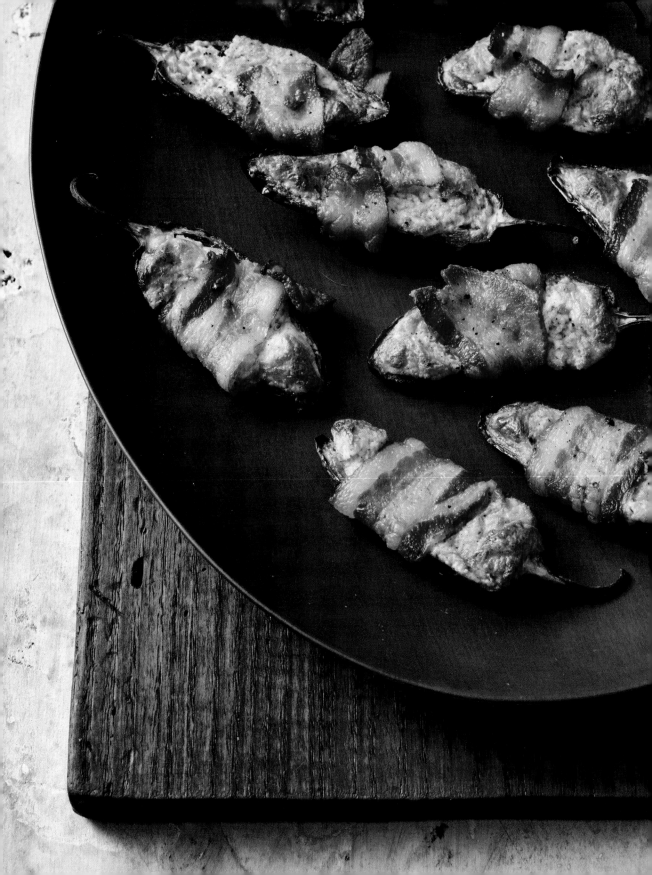

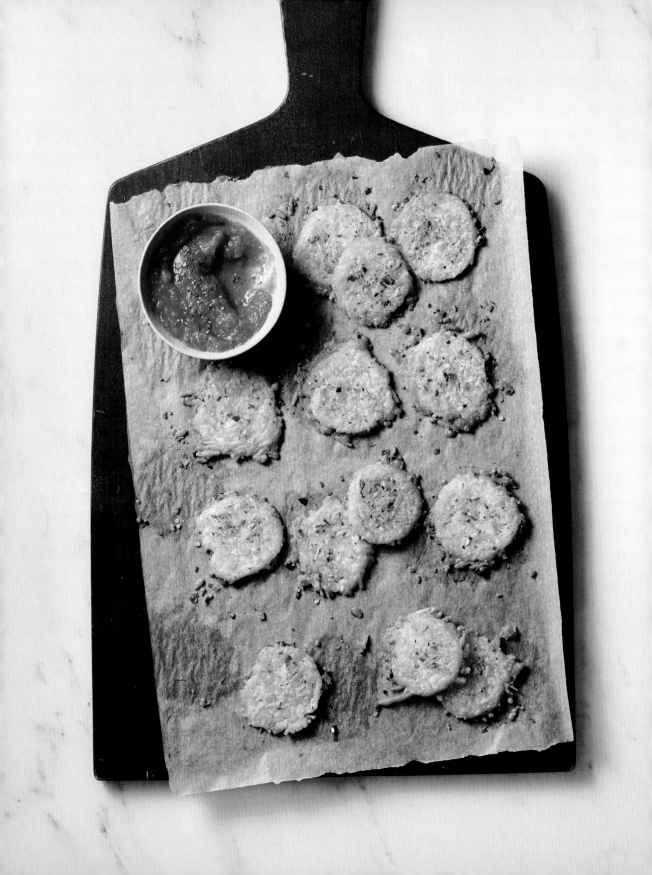

HERBED PARMESAN CRISPS

PREP TIME: 5 MINUTES ★ COOK TIME: 8 MINUTES ★ MAKES: 12 (3 CRISPS PER SERVING) ★ SERVINGS: 4

A common complaint on keto diets is "I miss potato chips and nacho chips." Well, complain no more! Cheese can be baked into crispy carb-free chips in no time at all. You'll never crave high-carb processed snack foods again!

¼ teaspoon garlic powder

¼ teaspoon dried oregano

¼ teaspoon dried thyme

¼ teaspoon red pepper flakes (optional)

Pinch of freshly ground black pepper

1¼ cups shredded Parmesan cheese

½ cup low-carb marinara sauce (optional), warmed, for dipping

1. Preheat the oven to 400°F. Line two baking sheets with parchment paper.

2. In a small bowl, combine the garlic powder, oregano, thyme, pepper flakes (if using), and black pepper. Using a 1-tablespoon measure, place the Parmesan in 12 small tight piles 2 inches apart on the prepared baking sheets. Sprinkle the tops with the spice mixture.

3. Transfer to the oven and bake until set and golden on the edges, 6 to 8 minutes, turning the baking sheets around halfway through baking.

4. Allow to cool on the pans for 1 minute. Remove to a plate lined with paper towels to cool completely. If desired, serve with marinara sauce (no sugar added) for dipping.

TIP: There are so many different spices and toppings for these crisps. Try mixing in or topping with your favorite seeds, spices, herbs, and even sliced jalapeños or pepperoni—they can never be boring. And you can also switch up the cheese and use your favorite hard grating cheese.

PER SERVING ★ CALORIES: 133 ★ GRAMS OF PROTEIN: 12 ★ GRAMS OF FAT: 8 ★ GRAMS OF CARBOHYDRATE: 2 ★ PERCENT OF PROTEIN: 36% ★ PERCENT OF FAT: 60% ★ PERCENT OF CARBOHYDRATE: 4%

GUACAMOLE WITH PEPITAS AND POMEGRANATE

PREP TIME: 5 MINUTES ★ SERVINGS: 4

There's nothing tastier than a good guac, right? I've added a few surprises like pumpkin seeds and pomegranate seeds to turn good to great. Forget high-carb nacho chips and substitute low-fat pork rinds for a smoky crunch.

1 avocado, halved and pitted

1 tablespoon finely chopped shallot

2 cloves garlic, minced

3 tablespoons chopped fresh cilantro

3 tablespoons fresh lime juice

½ teaspoon Celtic sea salt

¼ teaspoon freshly ground black pepper

2 tablespoons hulled pumpkin seeds (pepitas), toasted

2 tablespoons pomegranate seeds

2 ounces (4 small handfuls) pork rinds, for serving

1. Scoop the avocado into a bowl (or a large mortar). Add the shallot, garlic, cilantro, lime juice, sea salt, and pepper and use a potato masher (or the pestle) to mash until combined, but the avocado should still be a little chunky. (If not serving right away, refrigerate, but sprinkle with some lemon juice to keep the guacamole from turning brown.)

2. Garnish with the toasted pepitas and pomegranate seeds. Serve with the pork rinds.

PER SERVING ★ CALORIES: 195 ★ GRAMS OF PROTEIN: 12 ★ GRAMS OF FAT: 14 ★ GRAMS OF CARBOHYDRATE: 8 ★ PERCENT OF PROTEIN: 23% ★ PERCENT OF FAT: 61% ★ PERCENT OF CARBOHYDRATE: 16%

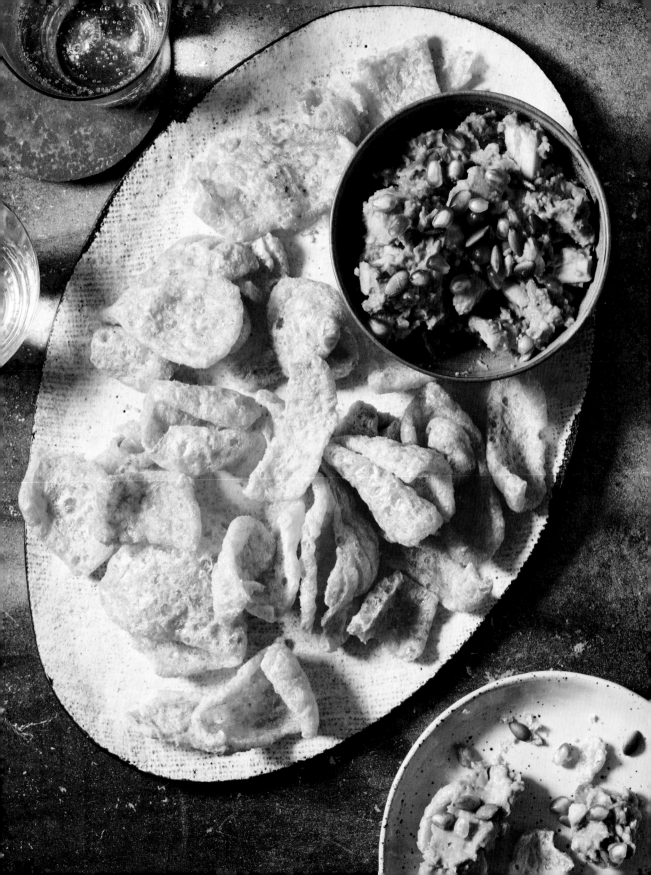

SPINACH AND ARTICHOKE DIP

PREP TIME: 10 MINUTES ★ COOK TIME: 30 MINUTES ★ SERVINGS: 6 (¼ TO ⅓ CUP PER SERVING)

Everyone gravitates toward this classic comfort food dip at parties, and it's gone before you know it. Now you can enjoy this appetizer without guilt while keto-ing your way to a lean, trim body.

1 tablespoon extra-virgin olive oil

½ yellow onion, finely diced

2 cloves garlic, minced

½ teaspoon Celtic sea salt

¼ teaspoon cayenne pepper

¼ teaspoon freshly ground black pepper

4 ounces frozen chopped spinach, thawed and squeezed of excess liquid

4 ounces full-fat cream cheese, at room temperature

⅓ cup mayonnaise

¼ cup shredded Parmigiano-Reggiano cheese

1 cup grated low-moisture whole-milk mozzarella cheese

1 (14-ounce) can water-packed artichokes, drained, rinsed, and chopped

6 stalks celery, cut into thirds

½ English cucumber, cut into wheels

1. Preheat the oven to 400°F.

2. Heat a medium sauté pan over medium heat and add the olive oil. Add the onion and cook until softened, about 5 minutes. Add the garlic, sea salt, cayenne, and black pepper and cook an additional minute. Remove from the heat and allow to cool completely.

3. In a large bowl, combine the spinach, cream cheese, mayonnaise, Parmigiano, ⅔ cup of the mozzarella, the artichokes, and the cooled onion mixture and stir until combined.

4. Scoop the dip into a 1-quart baking dish. Sprinkle the remaining ⅓ cup mozzarella over the top of the dip. Bake until the top is golden brown and the dip is bubbling, 18 to 20 minutes.

5. Serve with the celery sticks and cucumber wheels.

PER SERVING ★ CALORIES: 284 ★ GRAMS OF PROTEIN: 9 ★ GRAMS OF FAT: 24 ★ GRAMS OF CARBOHYDRATE: 8 ★ PERCENT OF PROTEIN: 13% ★ PERCENT OF FAT: 76% ★ PERCENT OF CARBOHYDRATE: 11%

LUNCHES

If you're a lunch lover, welcome to the table. I've got an array of comfort-to-the-max dishes—all easy to make, and many can be packed up and taken to work.

One of my favorites is the Keto Comfort Bacon Burger—hey, isn't bacon the number one reason to go keto? There's a lot more, too—even recipes made with steak (at least the number two reason to follow a keto diet!).

ASIAN-MARINATED FLANK STEAK STIR-FRY

PREP TIME: 15 MINUTES + MARINATING TIME ★ COOK TIME: 17 MINUTES ★ SERVINGS: 4

Although I'm Italian, I grew up eating a lot of Chinese food, and I love it. You can often find me at my local Chinese eatery, where the waiters and the kitchen staff know my first, last, and middle names. It's easy to overeat this amazing food, so I have to exercise a bit of self-control, especially when keto dieting. One way I do that is by cooking keto-friendly stir-fry dishes like this one at home.

STEAK

⅓ cup coconut aminos

Juice of 2 limes

1-inch piece fresh ginger, thinly sliced

2 cloves garlic, thinly sliced

Celtic sea salt

Freshly ground black pepper

2 scallions, white and light-green parts only, thinly sliced

1½ pounds flank steak, trimmed

1 tablespoon extra-virgin olive oil

STIR-FRY

1 tablespoon toasted sesame oil

1 tablespoon coconut oil

1 cup small broccoli florets

1 cup cauliflower florets

2 scallions, white and light-green parts only, thinly sliced

1 tablespoon minced fresh ginger

1 clove garlic, minced

Celtic sea salt

Freshly ground black pepper

¼ teaspoon red pepper flakes

2 tablespoons coconut aminos

1 cup bean sprouts

FOR SERVING

1 tablespoon sesame seeds, toasted

2 tablespoons chopped fresh cilantro leaves

Lime wedges

PER SERVING ★ CALORIES: 295 ★ GRAMS OF PROTEIN: 38 ★ GRAMS OF FAT: 10 ★ GRAMS OF CARBOHYDRATE: 11 ★ PERCENT OF PROTEIN: 53% ★ PERCENT OF FAT: 32% ★ PERCENT OF CARBOHYDRATE: 15%

1. **PREPARE THE STEAK:** In a baking dish or large zip-top bag, combine the coconut aminos, lime juice, ginger, garlic, sea salt, pepper, scallions, and flank steak. Allow to marinate for 25 minutes at room temperature.

2. In a large cast-iron skillet or heavy-bottomed sauté pan, heat the olive oil over medium-high heat. Remove the steak from the marinade, add to the pan, discarding the marinade, and sear on both sides until medium-rare, 3 to 4 minutes per side. Remove to a plate to rest for 8 to 10 minutes while you make the stir-fry.

3. **PREPARE THE STIR-FRY:** In the same pan used to cook the steak, heat the sesame oil and coconut oil over high heat. Add the broccoli and cauliflower and cook until beginning to turn golden brown and tender, 5 to 7 minutes. Add the scallions, ginger, garlic, sea salt, pepper, and pepper flakes and cook for 1 minute, then add the coconut aminos and bean sprouts and cook 1 minute more.

4. Divide the stir-fry among 4 plates. Thinly slice the steak and lay the slices on top of the stir-fry. Sprinkle with sesame seeds and cilantro and serve with lime wedges.

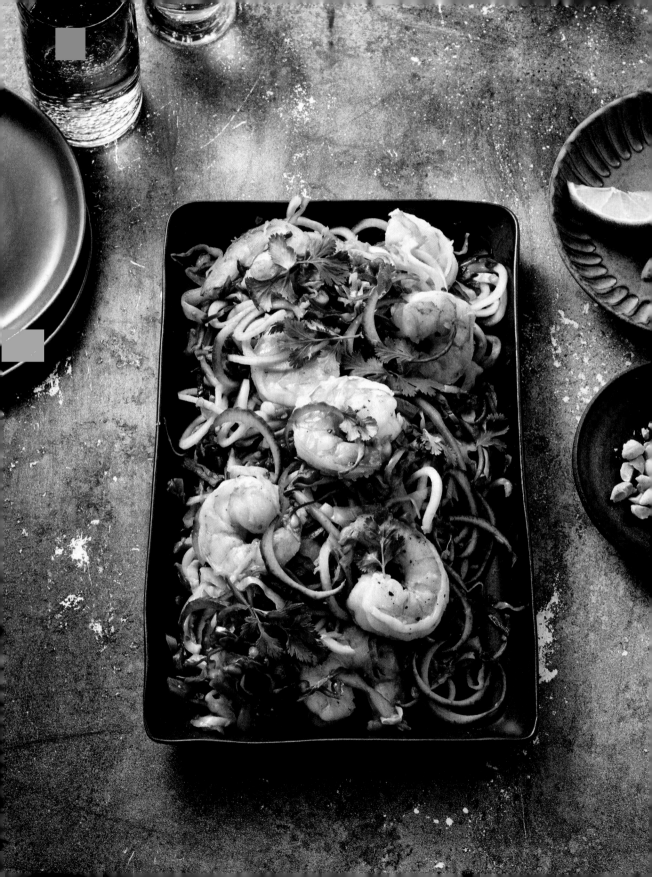

SHRIMP PAD THAI

PREP TIME: 20 MINUTES ★ COOK TIME: 15 MINUTES ★ SERVINGS: 4

I drew inspiration from Thailand to create my keto version of this country's popular street food. The star of the dish is its large delectable shrimp, surrounded by satisfying low-carb veggies tossed in Asian flavors. If this is an ethnic dish you love, please learn to make it at home. At most restaurants, a serving of Pad Thai weighs in at 1,000 to 1,500 calories and loads you up with carby noodles and about a three-day supply of salt.

1 tablespoon toasted sesame oil

2 tablespoons coconut oil

1 pound large shrimp, peeled and deveined, tails removed

Celtic sea salt

Freshly ground black pepper

2 scallions, white and light-green parts only, minced

3 cloves garlic, minced

1-inch piece fresh ginger, peeled and minced

1½ cups thinly sliced green cabbage

1½ cups thinly sliced red cabbage

3 tablespoons coconut aminos

2 tablespoons creamy unsweetened natural peanut butter

2 tablespoons fresh lime juice, plus wedges for serving

1 tablespoon fish sauce

½ English cucumber, spiralized into noodles

2 tablespoons fresh cilantro, for garnish

⅓ cup salted, roasted peanuts, chopped, for garnish

Lime wedges, for serving

1. Heat a large heavy-bottomed sauté pan over medium-high heat and add the sesame oil and coconut oil. Season the shrimp with salt and pepper. Add to the pan and cook until pink and opaque, about 2 minutes per side. Remove to a plate using a slotted spoon and set aside.

2. Add the scallions, garlic, and ginger to the pan and cook for 1 minute. Add the cabbage and cook until wilted and tender, 5 to 7 minutes. Add the coconut aminos, peanut butter, lime juice, and fish sauce and toss to combine.

3. Remove from the heat. Add the cucumber noodles and cooked shrimp and toss to combine. Sprinkle with the cilantro and chopped peanuts and serve with lime wedges.

PER SERVING ★ CALORIES: 302 ★ GRAMS OF PROTEIN: 29 ★ GRAMS OF FAT: 14 ★ GRAMS OF CARBOHYDRATE: 17 ★ PERCENT OF PROTEIN: 38% ★ PERCENT OF FAT: 41% ★ PERCENT OF CARBOHYDRATE: 21%

CAJUN FISH "TACOS"

PREP TIME: 20 MINUTES ★ COOK TIME: 8 MINUTES ★ SERVINGS: 4

Who eats tacos on a diet? You do! The "taco" here is a big crunchy Bibb lettuce leaf. You won't miss the real thing, because with tacos it's all about the spicy filling.

¼ cup mayonnaise

2 tablespoons fresh lime juice

¼ teaspoon ground cumin

2 tablespoons fresh cilantro leaves, chopped, plus more for garnish

Pinch of cayenne pepper

Celtic sea salt

Freshly ground black pepper

1 cup thinly sliced red cabbage

2 tablespoons extra-virgin olive oil

1½ pounds skinless cod fillet, cut into 2-inch pieces

2 tablespoons Cajun Spice Blend (recipe follows)

12 large green Bibb leaves

Lime wedges, for serving

1. In a large bowl, combine the mayonnaise, lime juice, cumin, cilantro, cayenne, and salt and black pepper to taste. Add the red cabbage and toss to coat. Set aside for 10 minutes to marinate.

2. Meanwhile, in a large cast-iron skillet or heavy-bottomed sauté pan, heat the olive oil over medium-high heat. Evenly sprinkle the fish on both sides with the Cajun spice blend. Add the fish to the pan and sear on both sides until cooked through and fragrant, about 4 minutes per side.

3. Divide the fish evenly among the Bibb lettuce leaves and top with equal amounts of the cabbage slaw. Sprinkle with additional cilantro leaves on top and serve with lime wedges.

PER SERVING ★ CALORIES: 316 ★ GRAMS OF PROTEIN: 27 ★ GRAMS OF FAT: 20 ★ GRAMS OF CARBOHYDRATE: 7 ★ PERCENT OF PROTEIN: 34% ★ PERCENT OF FAT: 57% ★ PERCENT OF CARBOHYDRATE: 9%

CAJUN SPICE BLEND

MAKES ABOUT 5 TABLESPOONS

1 tablespoon sweet paprika

1 tablespoon garlic powder

1½ teaspoons dried oregano

1½ teaspoons dried thyme

1½ teaspoons freshly ground black pepper

1 teaspoon cayenne pepper

1 teaspoon onion powder

1 teaspoon Celtic sea salt

Combine all of the ingredients and store in an airtight container.

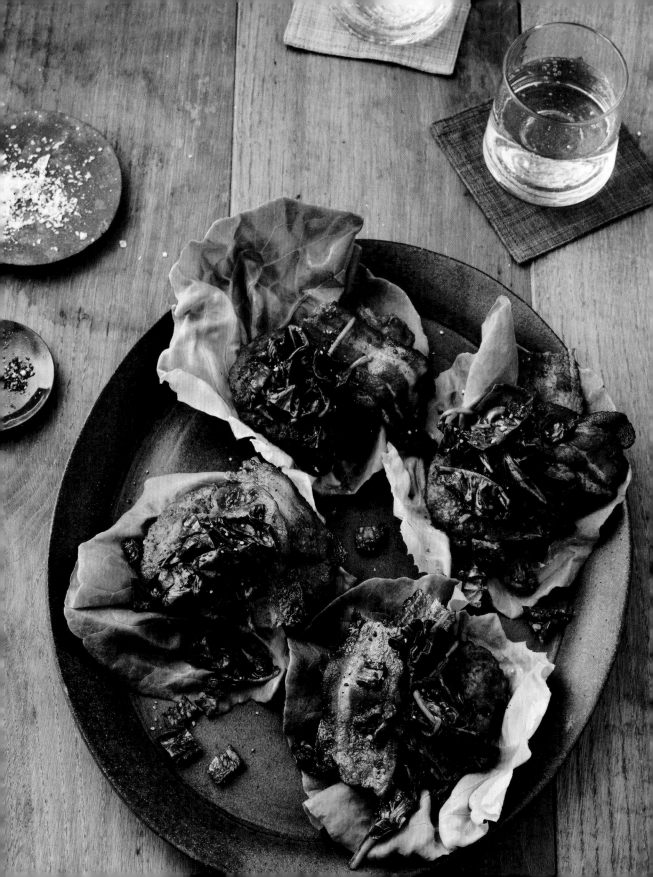

KETO COMFORT BACON BURGER

PREP TIME: 15 MINUTES ★ COOK TIME: 17 MINUTES, INCLUDING 5 MINUTES TO PAN-FRY THE BACON ★ SERVINGS: 4

Have you ever said to yourself, "A juicy burger sounds good right now"? Before you make a run to your nearest fast-food joint, try this version of a delish bacon burger. In the time it takes to get to the drive-through, you'll have this served up on your plate. I promise it will satisfy your cravings for a junk burger.

1½ pounds ground beef

2 teaspoons garlic powder

2 teaspoons onion powder

1 teaspoon sweet paprika

1 teaspoon Celtic sea salt

¼ teaspoon freshly ground black pepper

1 tablespoon extra-virgin olive oil

4 cups fresh spinach

Olive oil or avocado oil cooking spray

Bibb lettuce or large collard green leaves (midrib removed)

4 tablespoons oil-packed sun-dried tomatoes, whole

4 slices bacon, cooked to crisp and cut in half

1. In a medium bowl, mix together the beef, garlic powder, onion powder, paprika, sea salt, and pepper, combining with your hands until well blended. Form into 4 equal-sized patties. Set aside.

2. In a small skillet, heat the olive oil over medium heat. Add the spinach and sauté until just wilted. Remove from the skillet and set aside.

3. Coat a sauté pan generously with cooking spray. Cook the burgers over medium-high heat on both sides until cooked through, 5 to 6 minutes per side. Drain the burgers on a plate lined with paper towels.

4. Place each burger on top of a large leaf. Dividing evenly, top with the spinach, sun-dried tomatoes, and bacon. Wrap the burgers in the leaves and enjoy them "bunless."

PER SERVING ★ CALORIES: 400 ★ GRAMS OF PROTEIN: 26 ★ GRAMS OF FAT: 33 ★ GRAMS OF CARBOHYDRATE: 6 ★ PERCENT OF PROTEIN: 20% ★ PERCENT OF FAT: 74% ★ PERCENT OF CARBOHYDRATE: 6%

MEDITERRANEAN SALMON BURGER

PREP TIME: 15 MINUTES + 15 MINUTES REFRIGERATION ★ COOK TIME: 10 MINUTES ★ SERVINGS: 4

Tasty ingredients put together well—that's how I describe this wonderful salmon burger. It will land you immediately into your food-comfort zone.

SALMON BURGERS

1 pound skinless wild salmon fillet

½ cup almond flour

1 large egg

⅓ cup crumbled feta cheese

3 tablespoons minced red onion

2 tablespoons chopped, pitted Kalamata olives

1 tablespoon chopped fresh dill

1 tablespoon chopped fresh parsley

Grated zest and juice of 1 lemon

½ teaspoon ground coriander

Celtic sea salt

Freshly ground black pepper

MINTY YOGURT SAUCE

½ cup whole-milk plain Greek yogurt

3 tablespoons finely chopped English cucumber

1 tablespoon chopped fresh mint

1 tablespoon thinly sliced fresh chives

1 tablespoon extra-virgin olive oil

Juice of 1 lemon

Celtic sea salt

Freshly ground black pepper

FOR SERVING

Olive oil or avocado oil cooking spray

1 head Bibb lettuce, leaves separated

Dill sprigs, for garnish

1. MAKE THE SALMON BURGERS: In a food processor, pulse the salmon until it is the size of panko bread crumbs. Transfer to a bowl and add the almond flour, egg, feta, onion, olives, dill, parsley, lemon zest, lemon juice, coriander, and salt and pepper to taste. Form into 4 patties (about ¾ inch thick) and refrigerate for 15 minutes.

PER SERVING ★ CALORIES: 371 ★ GRAMS OF PROTEIN: 34 ★ GRAMS OF FAT: 23 ★ GRAMS OF CARBOHYDRATE: 7 ★ PERCENT OF PROTEIN: 36% ★ PERCENT OF FAT: 56% ★ PERCENT OF CARBOHYDRATE: 8%

2. **MEANWHILE, MAKE THE YOGURT SAUCE:** In a small bowl, combine the yogurt, cucumber, mint, chives, olive oil, lemon juice, and salt and pepper to taste.

3. **WHEN READY TO SERVE:** Coat a sauté pan generously with cooking spray. Add the salmon burgers and cook over medium-high heat until golden brown on both sides, 2 to 3 minutes per side.

4. Serve the salmon burgers on top of Bibb lettuce leaves and top with yogurt sauce. Garnish with dill sprigs.

TUNA SALAD OVER BIBB

PREP TIME: 10 MINUTES ★ SERVINGS: 4

If you're looking for comfort, look no further than tuna salad. This gift from the sea is loaded with omega-3 fatty acids that boost your mood, among other healthy actions. This tuna salad strikes a savory note atop a bed of crunchy Bibb lettuce.

4 (5-ounce) cans water-packed light tuna, drained

½ cup mayonnaise

1 tablespoon Dijon mustard

Juice of 1 lemon

¼ cup pitted, chopped Kalamata olives

1 shallot, finely chopped

2 tablespoons chopped fresh dill, plus more for garnish

2 tablespoons chopped fresh parsley

¼ teaspoon sweet paprika

Celtic sea salt and freshly ground black pepper

1 head Bibb lettuce, separated into leaves, for serving

In a large bowl, combine the tuna, mayo, mustard, lemon juice, olives, shallot, dill, parsley, paprika, and salt and pepper to taste and stir gently to combine. Divide the Bibb lettuce leaves among 4 plates. Dividing evenly, top with the tuna salad and garnish with dill.

PER SERVING ★ CALORIES: 393 ★ GRAMS OF PROTEIN: 37 ★ GRAMS OF FAT: 23 ★ GRAMS OF CARBOHYDRATE: 4 ★ PERCENT OF PROTEIN: 38% ★ PERCENT OF FAT: 53% ★ PERCENT OF CARBOHYDRATE: 9%

STEAK FAJITA PLATTER WITH PEPPERS AND AVOCADO MASH

PREP TIME: 35 MINUTES ★ COOK TIME: 15 MINUTES ★ SERVINGS: 4

Can you eat fajitas without tortillas? Yes, you can—this platter is so full of sizzling goodness you won't even miss them.

1 pound skirt steak, trimmed

Olive oil or avocado oil cooking spray

Celtic sea salt

Freshly ground black pepper

1 red bell pepper, cut into strips

1 yellow bell pepper, cut into strips

½ red onion, cut into ½-inch-thick wedges

1 tablespoon extra-virgin olive oil

1 teaspoon chili powder

1 teaspoon ground cumin

AVOCADO MASH

2 avocados, halved and pitted

¼ cup chopped fresh cilantro leaves

2 tablespoons fresh lime juice

Celtic sea salt

Freshly ground black pepper

1. Allow the steak to sit at room temperature for 20 minutes.

2. Coat a grill, grill pan, or large cast-iron skillet with cooking spray. Heat over medium-high heat. Season the steak with salt and black pepper. Cook for 3 to 4 minutes per side for medium-rare.

3. Remove to a board and allow to rest for 10 minutes.

4. Meanwhile, in a bowl, combine the bell peppers, onion, olive oil, chili powder, cumin, and salt and black pepper to taste. Toss to evenly coat.

5. Place the pepper/onion mixture on the grill or in the skillet and cook until charred and almost tender, 5 to 7 minutes.

6. MAKE THE AVOCADO MASH: Scoop the avocados into a medium bowl. Add the cilantro and lime juice and mash with a potato masher or the back of a fork until combined. Season with salt and pepper to taste.

7. When ready to serve, thinly slice the beef against the grain. Serve with the pepper/onion mixture and avocado mash.

PER SERVING ★ CALORIES: 395 ★ GRAMS OF PROTEIN: 26 ★ GRAMS OF FAT: 27 ★ GRAMS OF CARBOHYDRATE: 16 ★ PERCENT OF PROTEIN: 25% ★ PERCENT OF FAT: 60% ★ PERCENT OF CARBOHYDRATE: 15%

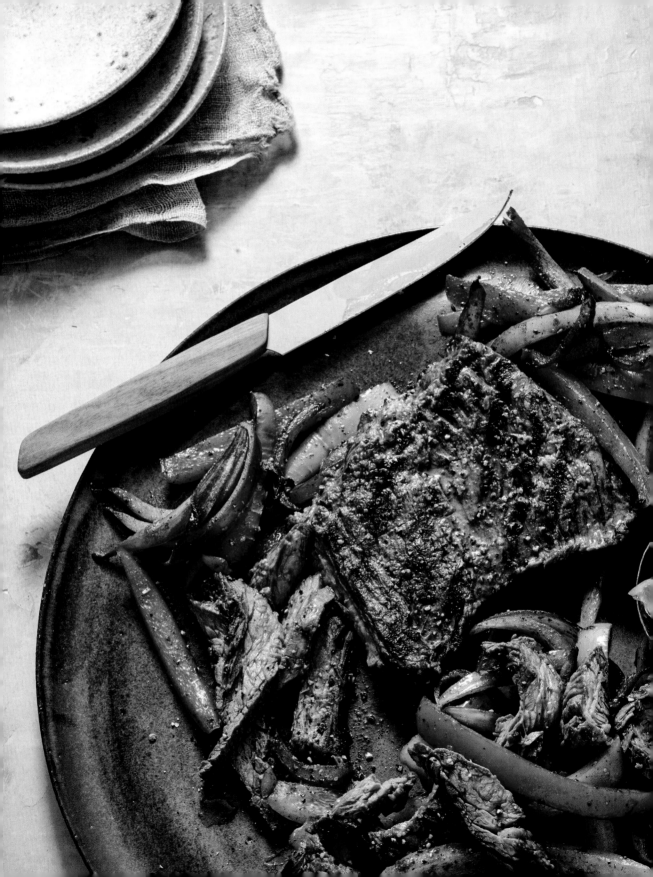

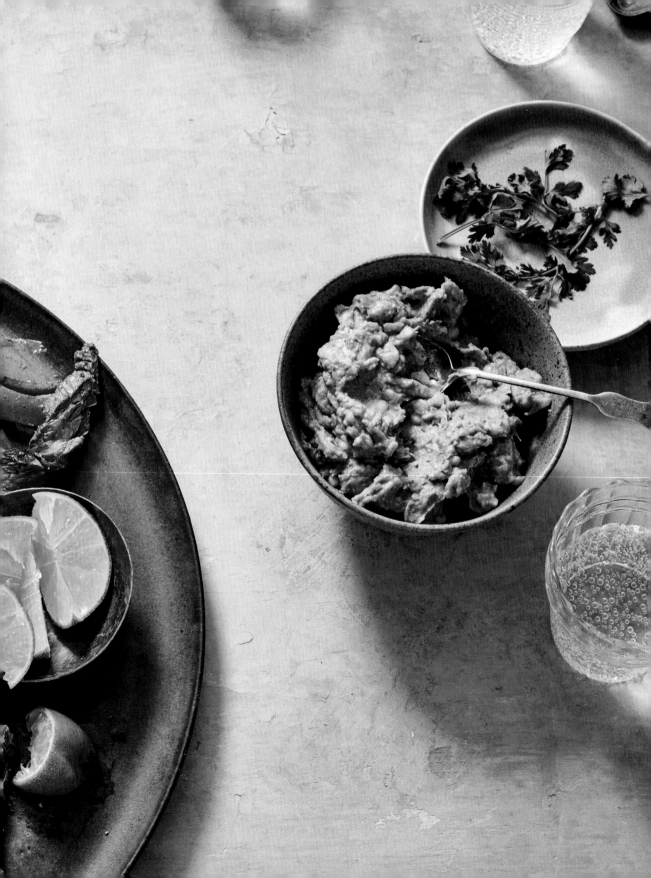

PORK FRIED RICE

PREP TIME: 10 MINUTES ★ COOK TIME: 17 MINUTES ★ SERVINGS: 4

Riced cauliflower is the keto vegetable du jour. I rarely eat regular rice anymore, because cauliflower rice actually tastes better to me.

1 head cauliflower, cut into small florets (see Tip)

2 tablespoons coconut oil

1 tablespoon toasted sesame oil

½ pound ground pork

Celtic sea salt

Freshly ground black pepper

2 cloves garlic, minced

2 scallions, white and light-green parts only, thinly sliced

1-inch piece fresh ginger, peeled and minced

2 heads baby bok choy, thinly sliced (about 1½ cups)

3 large eggs, beaten

2 tablespoons coconut aminos

1 tablespoon chili-garlic sauce

3 tablespoons chopped fresh cilantro

Lime wedges, for serving

1. In a food processor, pulse the cauliflower florets until they resemble rice. Set aside.

2. In a large nonstick sauté pan, heat both oils over medium-high heat. Add the pork and cook until browned on one side, about 5 minutes. Break the pork up with the back of a wooden spoon into crumbles and continue cooking another 4 minutes, until the pork is brown and cooked through. Season with salt and pepper to taste. Remove to a plate lined with paper towels.

3. Add the garlic, scallions, and ginger to the pan and cook for 1 minute. Add the bok choy and cauliflower rice and cook until tender, about 5 minutes. Season with salt and pepper.

4. Return the pork to the pan; stir it to combine with the other ingredients. Make a well in the center of the mixture. Add the eggs and allow to set for 2 minutes in the center of the pan. Break the eggs up and stir to evenly combine with the ingredients in the pan. Add the coconut aminos, chili-garlic sauce, and cilantro during the last minute of cooking. Serve with lime wedges.

TIP: If you don't like the labor of making your own cauliflower rice, you can buy it in the frozen vegetable section at most supermarkets. You'll need 4 cups here.

PER SERVING ★ CALORIES: 360 ★ GRAMS OF PROTEIN: 19 ★ GRAMS OF FAT: 24 ★ GRAMS OF CARBOHYDRATE: 16 ★ PERCENT OF PROTEIN: 22% ★ PERCENT OF FAT: 60% ★ PERCENT OF CARBOHYDRATE: 18%

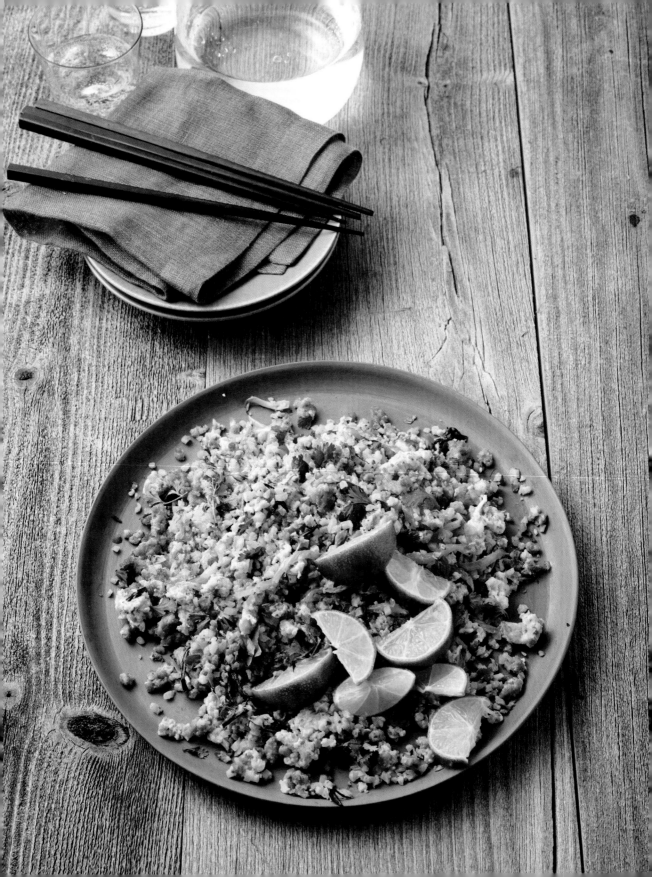

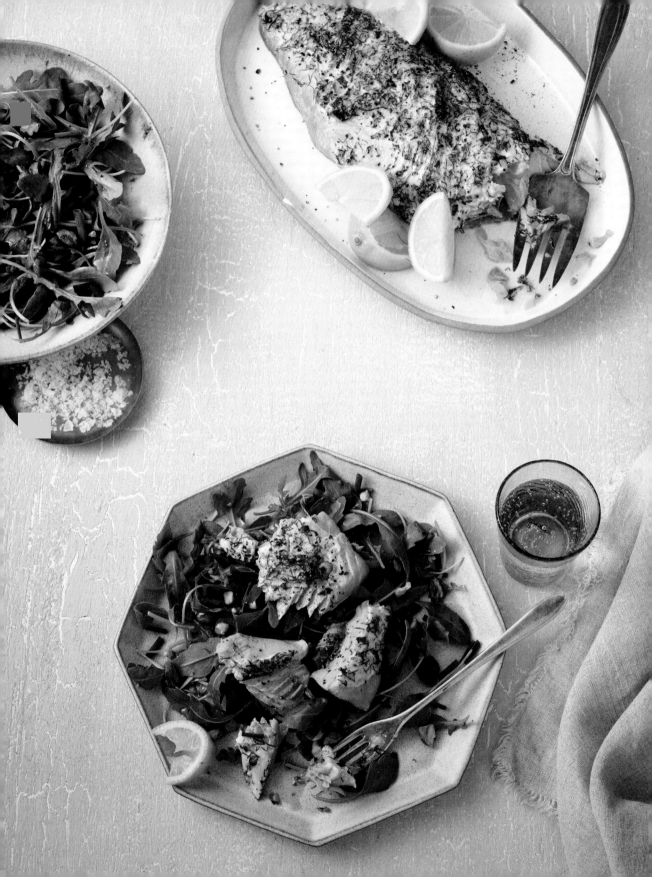

HERB AND GARLIC SALMON OVER ARUGULA

PREP TIME: 10 MINUTES ★ COOK TIME: 12 MINUTES ★ SERVINGS: 4

Salmon is packed with omega-3 fatty acids that are good for your heart and may protect against Alzheimer's disease. Make sure your salmon is wild-caught and not farm-raised. Otherwise, you might consume too many environmental toxins.

1 pound skin-on wild salmon fillets, pin bones removed

¼ cup mayonnaise

¼ cup chopped fresh dill

¼ cup chopped fresh parsley

2 cloves garlic, grated

Grated zest of ½ lemon and juice of 1 lemon

Celtic sea salt

Freshly ground black pepper

2 tablespoons extra-virgin olive oil

1 (5-ounce) container baby arugula

¼ cup (½-inch) pieces fresh chives

¼ cup pistachios, toasted

¼ cup pomegranate seeds

1. Preheat the oven to 400°F. Line a baking sheet with foil.

2. Arrange the salmon on the baking sheet. In a medium bowl, combine the mayonnaise, dill, parsley, garlic, and lemon zest. Season with salt and pepper to taste. Spread the mixture over the salmon fillets and bake until opaque and cooked to your liking, 10 to 12 minutes.

3. Meanwhile, in a small bowl, whisk together the lemon juice, olive oil, and salt and pepper to taste. In a large bowl, combine the arugula, chives, pistachios, and pomegranate seeds. Drizzle the dressing around the rim of the bowl and toss to evenly coat.

4. Serve the salmon atop a bed of the arugula.

PER SERVING ★ CALORIES: 421 ★ GRAMS OF PROTEIN: 26 ★ GRAMS OF FAT: 33 ★ GRAMS OF CARBOHYDRATE: 6 ★ PERCENT OF PROTEIN: 25% ★ PERCENT OF FAT: 70% ★ PERCENT OF CARBOHYDRATE: 5%

CHICKEN AND CAULIFLOWER TIKKA MASALA

PREP TIME: 15 MINUTES ★ COOK TIME: 25 MINUTES ★ SERVINGS: 4

Tikka masala is a popular dish of chunks of chicken in a creamy Indian-spiced sauce. Enjoy this flavorful keto version!

1 tablespoon garam masala

1 teaspoon ground cumin

1 teaspoon ground turmeric

¼ teaspoon cayenne pepper

1 tablespoon extra-virgin olive oil

¾ pound boneless, skinless chicken thighs, cut into 1-inch pieces

Celtic sea salt

Freshly ground black pepper

1 cup small cauliflower florets

½ yellow onion, finely diced

3 cloves garlic, minced

1-inch piece fresh ginger, peeled and minced

1 tablespoon tomato paste

1 cup full-fat unsweetened coconut milk

1 cup crushed canned tomatoes

¼ cup heavy cream

¼ cup chopped fresh cilantro

1. In a small bowl, combine the garam masala, cumin, turmeric, and cayenne and set aside.

2. In a large heavy-bottomed sauté pan with high sides, heat the olive oil over medium-high heat. Season the chicken with salt and black pepper, add to the pan, and sear on both sides until golden brown, about 4 minutes per side. Add the cauliflower florets during the last few minutes of cooking the chicken and cook until lightly golden, about 4 minutes.

3. Add the onion, garlic, and ginger and cook for another 2 minutes. Add the spice mixture and tomato paste and cook an additional minute. Add the coconut milk and tomatoes, scraping up any browned bits from the bottom of the pan. Allow to simmer for at least 8 and up to 10 minutes, until the sauce is thickened. Stir in the cream and sprinkle with the cilantro. Serve.

PER SERVING ★ CALORIES: 422 ★ GRAMS OF PROTEIN: 17 ★ GRAMS OF FAT: 34 ★ GRAMS OF CARBOHYDRATE: 13 ★ PERCENT OF PROTEIN: 16% ★ PERCENT OF FAT: 72% ★ PERCENT OF CARBOHYDRATE: 12%

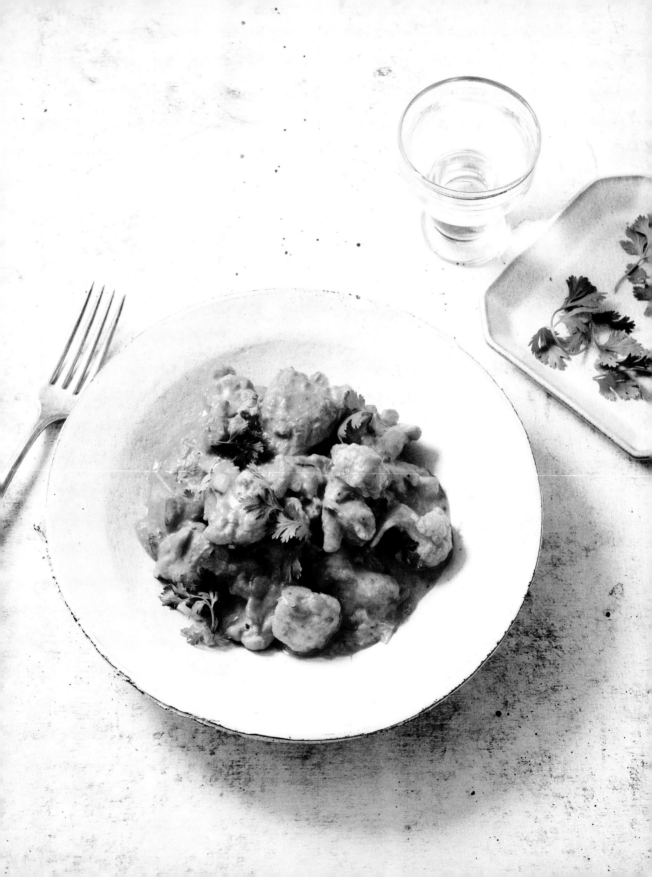

DINNERS

To say I merely love dinner is to say expensive champagne is just another something to satisfy your thirst. I don't just love it, I live for it. I love it because of the wonderful childhood memories I've experienced at the dinner table through the years.

But there's something I don't love about dinner as I've gotten older, and it's all those carbs and calories. They make you want to crash on the couch, loosen your belt, and doze off in a food coma.

So I worked very hard to remove the carbs and downsize the calories in our favorite comfort food dinners—and also keep them super delicious.

Check out all the entrées that follow, and choose those that appeal to you. Have a different one every day. Or, to save time through the week, cook in bulk and enjoy leftovers. The protein in most of these dishes is complemented by one or two nonstarchy vegetables for a complete, healthy meal.

MAMA'S KETO MEATBALLS WITH ZUCCHINI NOODLES

PREP TIME: 30 MINUTES ★ COOK TIME: 1½ HOURS (SEE TIP) ★ SERVINGS: 6

This dish is a keto version of my mother's signature dish, fondly known as Mama's Meatballs. While you won't find them on a mound of begging-to-be-twirled spaghetti, you'll still be wowed by their full-on flavor atop zoodles.

MARINARA SAUCE (SEE TIP)

1 tablespoon extra-virgin olive oil

1 clove garlic, crushed through a press

2 tablespoons finely chopped yellow onion

¾ teaspoon tomato paste

Red pepper flakes

Celtic sea salt

Freshly ground black pepper

1 (16-ounce) can tomato puree

½ (16-ounce) can crushed tomatoes

¼ cup chicken stock

1½ cups water

⅛ teaspoon liquid stevia (optional)

MEATBALLS

Olive oil or avocado oil cooking spray

⅓ cup chicken stock

¼ yellow onion, roughly chopped

1 clove garlic, peeled but whole

½ pound ground beef

½ pound ground pork

½ pound ground veal

⅓ cup crushed Herbed Parmesan Crisps (page 189) or store-bought Parmesan crisps (such as Whisps)

2 large eggs

¼ cup grated Parmigiano-Reggiano cheese

1 teaspoon red pepper flakes

¼ cup finely chopped fresh flat-leaf parsley

1 teaspoon Celtic sea salt

ZUCCHINI NOODLES

1 tablespoon extra-virgin olive oil

1 pound store-bought zucchini noodles

Celtic sea salt

Freshly ground black pepper

¼ cup grated Parmigiano-Reggiano cheese, for serving

1. MAKE THE MARINARA SAUCE: In a saucepot, heat the olive oil over medium-low heat. Add the garlic and onion and cook until the garlic is tender and the onion is

(recipe continues)

TIP: To shave over an hour off the cooking time, use a good-quality, low-carb store-bought marinara such as Rao's instead of the homemade.

translucent, about 5 minutes. Add the tomato paste and cook for 30 seconds. Season with red pepper flakes, salt, and black pepper to taste.

2. Add the tomato puree, crushed tomatoes, chicken stock, and water to the pot along with the liquid stevia (if using) and stir to combine. Bring to a simmer, season with salt to taste, cover, and simmer for 25 to 30 minutes. If the sauce is too thin, simmer uncovered for 2 to 3 minutes. If the sauce is too thick, add a little water. The sauce should be fairly thin and very smooth, but not watery.

3. MEANWHILE, MAKE THE MEATBALLS: Preheat the oven to 400°F. Coat a sheet pan with cooking spray.

4. In a food processor or blender, combine the chicken stock, onion, and garlic and puree. Transfer the mixture to a large bowl and add the meats, crisps, eggs, Parmigiano, pepper flakes, parsley, and salt. Mix with your hands until just combined, being careful not to overmix.

5. Grease your hands with olive oil and form the mixture into 12 balls a little smaller than golf balls.

6. Arrange the meatballs on the sheet pan and bake until browned, at least 18 and up to 20 minutes.

7. Transfer the finished meatballs to the marinara sauce and allow to simmer for 10 to 15 minutes.

8. PREPARE THE ZUCCHINI NOODLES: In a large sauté pan, heat the olive oil over medium-high heat until shimmering. Add the zucchini noodles and cook until tender but still a little crunchy, 2 to 3 minutes. Season with salt and black pepper to taste.

9. Serve the meatballs and sauce over the zucchini noodles sprinkled with the Parmigiano.

PER SERVING ★ CALORIES: 400 ★ GRAMS OF PROTEIN: 32 ★ GRAMS OF FAT: 21 ★ GRAMS OF CARBOHYDRATE: 20 ★ PERCENT OF PROTEIN: 32% ★ PERCENT OF FAT: 48% ★ PERCENT OF CARBOHYDRATE: 20%

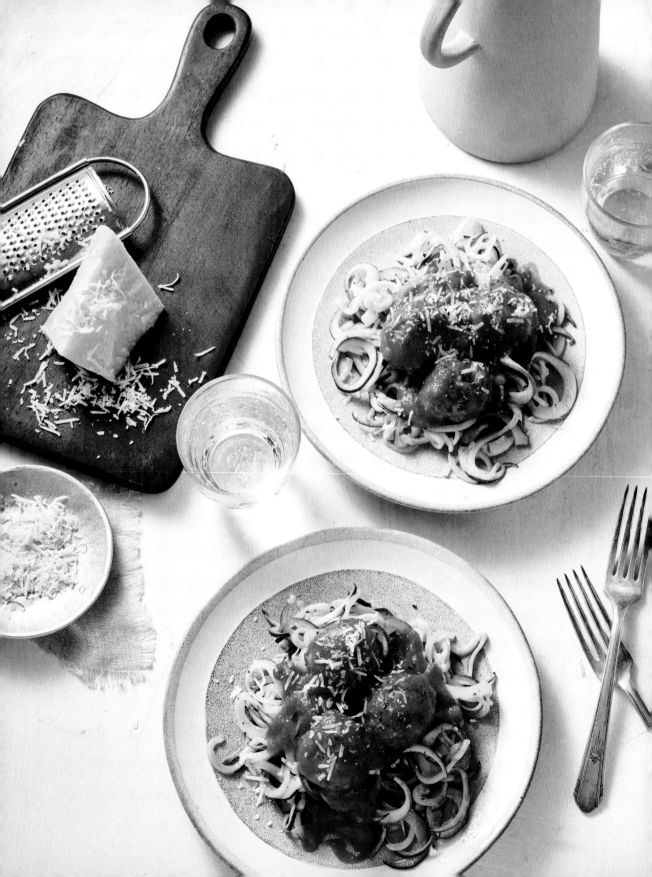

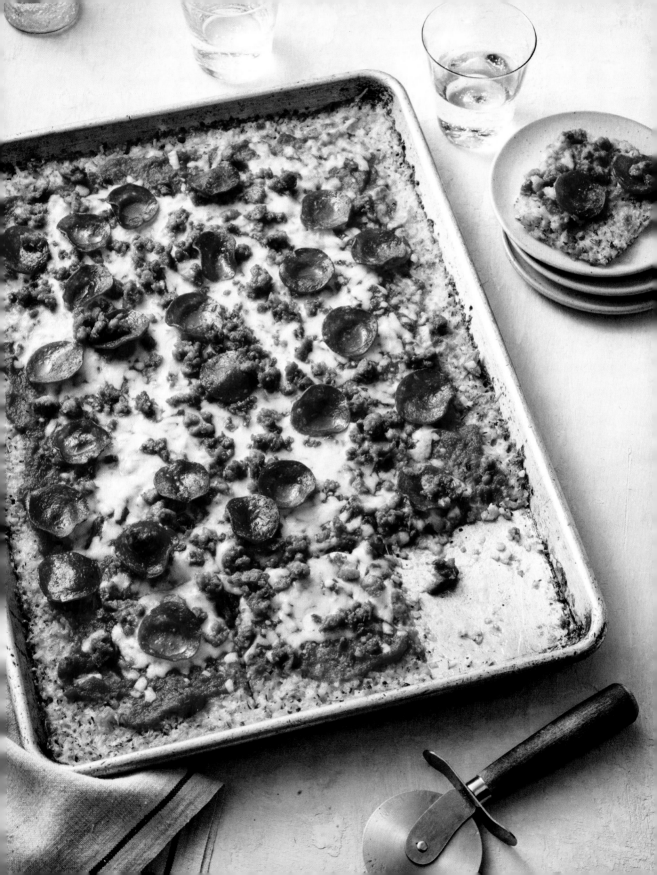

MEAT LOVERS' CAULIFLOWER PIZZA

PREP TIME: 15 MINUTES ★ COOK TIME: 35 MINUTES, INCLUDING 5 MINUTES TO PAN-FRY
THE SAUSAGE ★ SERVINGS: 4

When it comes to comfort foods, I love pizza! I could eat it hot
or cold, morning, noon, and night. If there was pizza-flavored
toothpaste, I'd eat it. But pizza is one of those foods with more
carbs than the carb police allow. So these days I make pizza with a
cauliflower crust. Not only is it virtually carb-free, it's also gluten-free.

CAULIFLOWER CRUST (SEE TIP)

1 tablespoon olive oil, for
greasing

2½ cups riced cauliflower
florets or store-bought
cauliflower rice

1 large egg, beaten

¾ cup grated Parmigiano-
Reggiano cheese

¾ cup grated low-moisture
whole-milk mozzarella cheese

½ teaspoon dried basil

½ teaspoon dried oregano

½ teaspoon dried thyme

Celtic sea salt

Freshly ground black pepper

TOPPINGS

¾ cup store-bought low-carb
marinara sauce (enough to
spread an even layer over the
crust)

¾ cup grated low-moisture
whole-milk mozzarella cheese

¼ cup pepperoni slices

2 links Italian sweet sausage,
casings removed, browned,
crumbled, and cooled

1. Preheat the oven to 425°F. Grease a baking sheet with
the olive oil and place in the oven to preheat.

2. **PREPARE THE CAULIFLOWER CRUST:** To make your own
cauliflower rice, place the florets in a food processor and
pulse until finely ground. Transfer the cauliflower rice to a
large bowl and cover with plastic wrap. Poke a hole in the
plastic wrap and microwave for 2 minutes until slightly
softened. Remove from the microwave and wring out any
excess liquid in a towel. (If using frozen cauliflower rice,
microwave it according to the package directions.)

3. Transfer the cauliflower rice to a bowl and add the
egg, Parmigano, mozzarella, basil, oregano, thyme, and
salt and pepper to taste. Remove the hot baking sheet

(recipe continues)

TIP: To save time, you can also buy prepared cauliflower pizza crusts in most grocery stores.

from the oven, being careful not to burn yourself. Spread the cauliflower mixture onto the hot pan with a silicone spatula to make a rectangle about ¼ inch thick. Return to the oven to bake until lightly golden brown, 15 to 18 minutes.

4. FOR THE TOPPINGS: Preheat the broiler to high.

5. Spread the sauce evenly over the top of the baked crust. Top with the mozzarella, pepperoni, and sausage. Return to the broiler until the cheese and pepperoni are lightly browned, 4 to 5 minutes, rotating the pan front to back halfway through. Allow to cool for 5 minutes before serving.

PER SERVING ★ CALORIES: 386 ★ GRAMS OF PROTEIN: 28 ★ GRAMS OF FAT: 26 ★ GRAMS OF CARBOHYDRATE: 10 ★ PERCENT OF PROTEIN: 29% ★ PERCENT OF FAT: 61% ★ PERCENT OF CARBOHYDRATE: 10%

HOT CRISPY KETO FRIED CHICKEN

PREP TIME: 15 MINUTES ★ COOK TIME: 15 MINUTES ★ SERVINGS: 4

On the Keto Comfort Food Diet, you will be boosting your dietary fat intake, but it's important not to go overboard. So when it came to the ultimate comfort food dinner—fried chicken—I had to be careful about not using too much fat. After experimenting a lot, I concluded that the amount of fat absorbed in frying is a function of time, not a function of the quantity of fat. I realized that if I fried chicken for a very short amount of time—a method called flash-frying—it would absorb very little fat but still achieve a crispy coating. Flash-frying lasts roughly 12 seconds at about 400°F, as opposed to 8 or 9 minutes for deep-frying at the same heat.

Grapeseed oil (about 2 quarts), for flash-frying

1 pound boneless, skinless chicken thighs

2 tablespoons + ¾ teaspoon adobo seasoning (such as Goya)

Celtic sea salt

Freshly ground black pepper

2 egg whites

1 cup almond flour

2½ tablespoons Hungarian sweet paprika

1. Pour 2 inches of oil into a large heavy pot that has at least a 6-quart capacity. Clip a deep-frying thermometer to the side of the pot and be sure the thermometer is not touching the bottom of the pot. Over medium heat, bring the oil temperature to 400°F.

2. Cut each chicken thigh into 4 or 5 even-sized chunks. Arrange all the chunks on a microwave-safe plate and season all over with ¾ teaspoon of the adobo seasoning, salt, and some pepper.

3. Place the plate in the microwave and cook for 1 minute 30 seconds. Remove the plate and turn each piece of chicken over. Microwave again until the chunks are just cooked through, another 1 to 2 minutes, depending on your microwave. Let the chicken cool to room temperature.

(recipe continues)

4. Set up a dredging station: Put the egg whites in a bowl and beat with a fork until just foamy, about 1 minute. In a separate wide and shallow bowl or a cake pan, combine the almond flour, paprika, and remaining 2 tablespoons adobo seasoning and mix thoroughly.

5. Submerge the chicken pieces in the egg whites. With a fork, toss to coat. One at a time, lift the chicken pieces from the egg whites, transfer to the almond flour mixture, and coat each piece thoroughly.

6. Set up a plate with a wire rack or paper towels on top and have it near the stove. Working in 4 batches, fry the chicken in the oil until deep golden brown, about 12 seconds. With metal tongs or a stainless steel spider basket, remove the chicken pieces and transfer to the rack or paper towels to drain off any excess oil. (Turn the stove off immediately after your last batch.)

PER SERVING ★ CALORIES: 360 ★ GRAMS OF PROTEIN: 22 ★ GRAMS OF FAT: 27 ★ GRAMS OF CARBOHYDRATE: 6 ★ PERCENT OF PROTEIN: 25% ★ PERCENT OF FAT: 68% ★ PERCENT OF CARBOHYDRATE: 7%

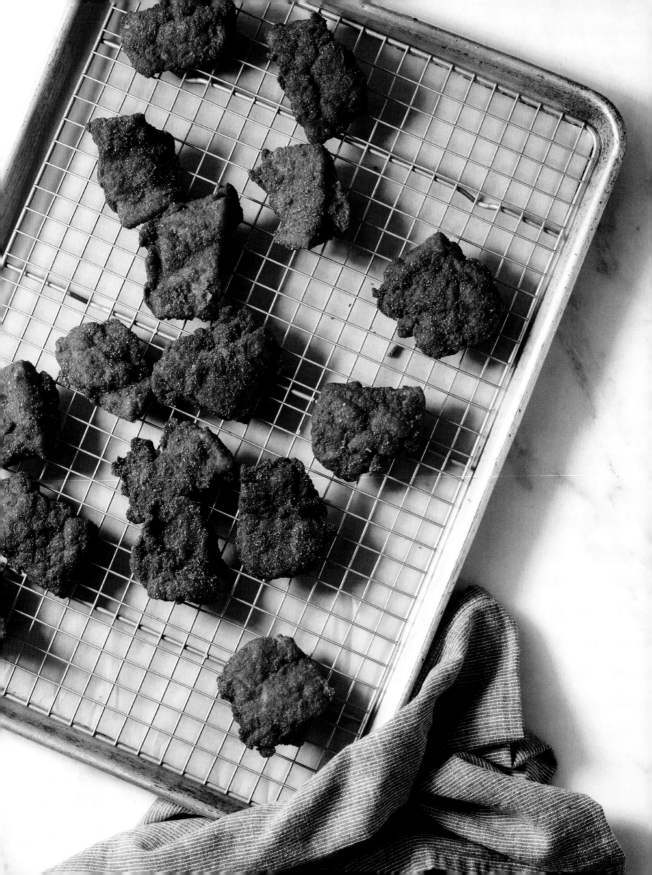

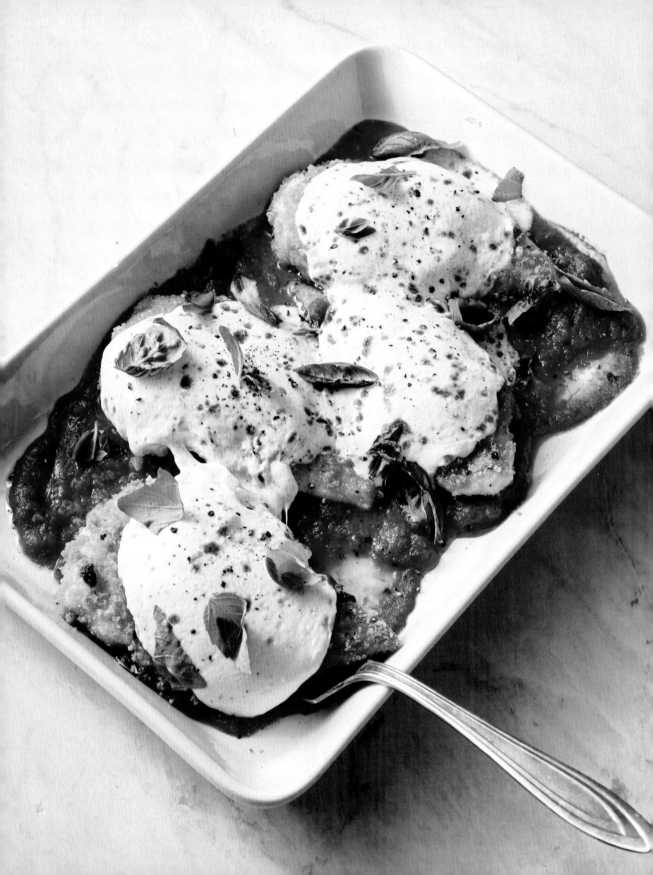

CHICKEN PARMESAN

PREP TIME: 15 MINUTES ★ COOK TIME: 25 MINUTES ★ SERVINGS: 4

Sometimes just a little innovation is all it takes to reinvent an old classic like Chicken Parmesan. I love a good chicken parm, and this is just as good as—even better than—its higher-carb counterpart.

Olive oil or avocado oil cooking spray

¾ cup almond flour

Celtic sea salt

Freshly ground black pepper

2 large eggs

2 (8-ounce) boneless, skinless chicken breasts, cut in half horizontally

2 cups store-bought good-quality low-carb marinara sauce, such as Rao's

4 ounces fresh whole-milk mozzarella cheese, cut into 8 even slices

¼ cup grated Parmigiano-Reggiano cheese

½ cup roughly chopped fresh basil leaves, for garnish

1. Preheat the broiler to high. Position a rack in the middle of the oven, about 18 inches below the broiler. Line a baking sheet with aluminum foil and spray with cooking spray.

2. Place the flour in a shallow dish and season with salt and pepper to taste.

3. Beat the eggs in a medium bowl.

4. One piece at a time, coat the chicken with egg, then move each cutlet to the flour mixture and coat evenly. Spray the chicken with 4 seconds of cooking spray and place on the prepared pan. Broil until browned on one side, about 8 minutes, then flip the chicken over and brown the other side.

5. Bring the marinara sauce to a simmer in a large saucepan.

6. Remove the chicken from the broiler and place it in a large baking dish. Top each piece of chicken with the marinara sauce and 2 slices of mozzarella.

7. Return the chicken to the broiler and cook until the cheese is melted. Remove from the broiler and sprinkle the Parmigiano evenly over the chicken. Garnish with the basil and serve.

PER SERVING ★ CALORIES: 400 ★ GRAMS OF PROTEIN: 48 ★ GRAMS OF FAT: 18 ★ GRAMS OF CARBOHYDRATE: 9 ★ PERCENT OF PROTEIN: 48% ★ PERCENT OF FAT: 41% ★ PERCENT OF CARBOHYDRATE: 11%

SHRIMP AND CHEESY CAULIFLOWER GRITS

PREP TIME: 15 MINUTES ★ COOK TIME: 25 MINUTES ★ SERVINGS: 6

It's rice . . . it's pizza crust . . . it's cauliflower grits! Cauliflower has emerged as a superhero veggie because you can use it in so many ways—especially as a sub for carbs.

CHEDDAR GRITS

1 small head cauliflower, cut into florets

2 tablespoons unsalted grass-fed butter

⅓ cup chicken stock

Celtic sea salt

Freshly ground black pepper

1 cup grated sharp cheddar cheese

SHRIMP

6 slices bacon, chopped

3 scallions, white and light-green parts only, chopped

1 green bell pepper, finely diced

2 cloves garlic, minced

Pinch of cayenne pepper

Celtic sea salt

Freshly ground black pepper

1½ pounds medium-large shrimp, peeled and deveined

½ cup chicken stock

2 tablespoons fresh lemon juice

FOR SERVING

2 scallions, thinly sliced, for garnish

Hot sauce

1. MAKE THE CHEDDAR GRITS: In a food processor, pulse the cauliflower florets until they resemble grits (about 3 cups total; if you have more than you need, refrigerate it for another use).

2. Heat a large sauté pan over medium-high heat and add the butter. Add the cauliflower grits and cook for 3 minutes, until the cauliflower is tender. Add the chicken stock and cook until creamy, another 2 to 3 minutes. Season with salt and pepper to taste. Stir in the cheddar and allow to melt.

3. MAKE THE SHRIMP: Lay the bacon in a cold skillet and place over medium-high heat. Allow to cook until browned and crispy, 6 to 7 minutes. With a slotted spoon, remove the bacon to a plate lined with paper towels.

4. Add the scallions, bell pepper, and garlic to the pan and cook until softened, 5 to 6 minutes. Season with the cayenne and salt and black pepper to taste.

5. Season the shrimp with salt and black pepper. Add to the sauté pan and cook until pink and opaque on both sides, about 2 minutes per side. During the last 2 minutes of cooking, add the chicken stock, lemon juice, and bacon. Allow to simmer until combined.

6. TO SERVE: Spoon the shrimp over the cheesy cauliflower grits. Sprinkle with the sliced scallions and serve with hot sauce.

PER SERVING ★ CALORIES: 316 ★ GRAMS OF PROTEIN: 34 ★ GRAMS OF FAT: 17 ★ GRAMS OF CARBOHYDRATE: 6 ★ PERCENT OF PROTEIN: 43% ★ PERCENT OF FAT: 49% ★ PERCENT OF CARBOHYDRATE: 8%

EGGPLANT LASAGNA WITH BEEF

PREP TIME: 25 MINUTES ★ COOK TIME: 40 MINUTES ★ SERVINGS: 6

I love a rich rectangular slab of lasagna. But the problem is that this classic Italian dish is layered with high-carb noodles. Okay, this really isn't a "problem" anymore because I use strips of eggplant to substitute for the noodles. That way, you can enjoy a healthy, soul-satisfying lasagna with only a fraction of the carbs.

MEAT SAUCE

2 tablespoons extra-virgin olive oil

½ yellow onion, chopped

3 garlic cloves, minced

4 ounces ground chuck

Celtic sea salt

Freshly ground black pepper

1 cup torn basil

1 (28-ounce) can chopped tomatoes

Red pepper flakes

⅛ to ¼ teaspoon liquid stevia (optional), to taste

FOR ASSEMBLY

2 tablespoons extra-virgin olive oil

1 medium eggplant (1 pound 3 ounces), sliced lengthwise into ¼-inch-thick slabs (about 12 slices total)

Celtic sea salt

Freshly ground black pepper

1 cup whole-milk ricotta cheese

⅔ cup grated Parmigiano-Reggiano cheese

¾ cup grated low-moisture whole-milk mozzarella cheese

1. MAKE THE MEAT SAUCE: In a large sauté pan, heat the olive oil over medium-high heat. Add the onion and cook until it begins to become translucent, about 5 minutes. Add the garlic and cook an additional minute.

2. Season the ground beef with salt and black pepper. Add the beef to the pan, breaking it into smaller pieces. Brown the beef thoroughly, for 2 to 4 minutes, then break it into smaller pieces using a wooden spoon. Add half of the torn basil and all of the tomatoes. Season again with salt, black pepper, and pepper flakes to taste. If the sauce is still too bitter, add some liquid stevia. Bring the sauce to a simmer and cook for 1 minute. Set aside.

3. **TO ASSEMBLE:** Preheat the broiler to high. Line three baking sheets with foil and grease them with one-third of the olive oil.

4. Lay the eggplant slices on the baking sheets and season with salt and pepper. Brush the slices on both sides with another third of the olive oil. Broil the eggplant until slightly browned and almost tender, 6 to 8 minutes, flipping the slices halfway through. Remove and allow to cool.

5. Preheat the oven to 450°F. Grease an 8 x 8-inch baking dish with the remaining olive oil and set aside.

6. In a medium bowl, combine the ricotta and ⅓ cup of the Parmigiano. Season the cheese mixture with salt and pepper to taste.

7. Spread one-quarter of the sauce over the bottom of the prepared baking dish. Make a layer of the roasted eggplant on top of the sauce, covering the bottom of the dish. Spread another one-quarter of the sauce over the eggplant. Spread half of the ricotta mixture over the eggplant. Repeat with another layer of eggplant, another one-quarter of sauce, and the remaining ricotta mixture. Top with eggplant slices and spread the remaining sauce over the eggplant. Sprinkle the top of the lasagna with the mozzarella and remaining ⅓ cup Parmigiano.

8. Cover the baking dish with foil and bake for 15 minutes. Uncover and continue to bake until the cheese begins to brown, another 10 minutes. Let the lasagna rest for 5 minutes in order to release extra steam and allow the ingredients to set before serving. Garnish with the remaining basil.

PER SERVING ★ CALORIES: 385 ★ GRAMS OF PROTEIN: 20 ★ GRAMS OF FAT: 27 ★ GRAMS OF CARBOHYDRATE: 14 ★ PERCENT OF PROTEIN: 22% ★ PERCENT OF FAT: 63% ★ PERCENT OF CARBOHYDRATE: 15%

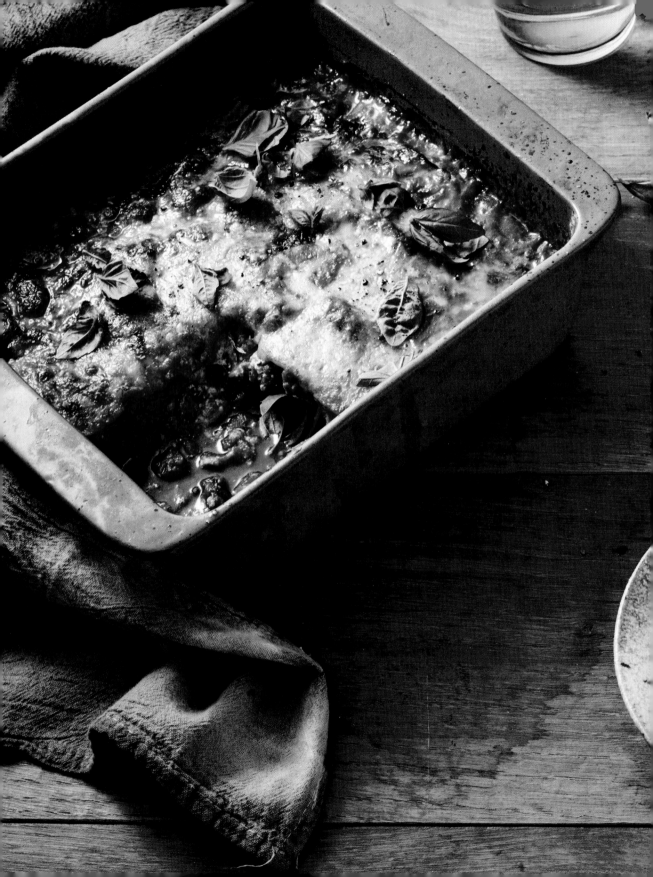

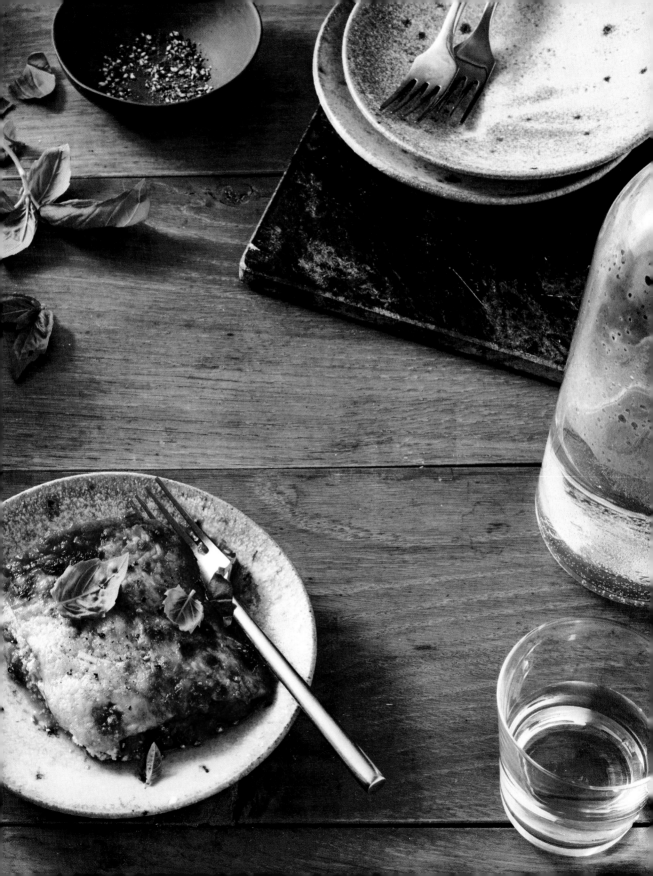

SLOPPY JOE POT PIE

PREP TIME: 15 MINUTES + 20 MINUTES REFRIGERATION ★ COOK TIME: 30 MINUTES ★ SERVINGS: 6

Here's a new twist on America's favorite hot sandwich, the Sloppy Joe, reincarnated as a hearty, comforting pot pie. By the way, there really was a "Joe" who invented the famous sandwich in the 1930s at his café in Sioux City, Iowa. Legend has it that he added tomato sauce to his meat sandwiches, and the rest is history. Was he sloppy? That I don't know!

SLOPPY JOE MIXTURE

2 tablespoons extra-virgin olive oil

2 cloves garlic

1 yellow onion, quartered

½ small green bell pepper, cut into large pieces

Celtic sea salt

Freshly ground black pepper

12 ounces ground beef

2 tablespoons coconut aminos

1 teaspoon chili powder

1 teaspoon sweet paprika

¾ cup tomato puree

½ cup water

1 tablespoon brown sugar erythritol

BISCUITS

¾ cup + 2 tablespoons almond flour

1½ teaspoons baking powder

¼ teaspoon Celtic sea salt

¼ teaspoon freshly ground black pepper

2 tablespoons cold unsalted grass-fed butter, cubed

1 large egg, beaten

¼ cup sour cream

1. PREPARE THE SLOPPY JOE MIXTURE: Heat a 12-inch cast-iron skillet over medium-high heat and add the olive oil. Add the garlic, onion, and bell pepper and cook until softened, about 5 minutes. Season with salt and black pepper to taste. Add the beef to the pan and cook, using a wooden spoon to break it into smaller pieces, until browned, 7 to 9 minutes. Add the coconut aminos, chili powder, and paprika and season with salt and black pepper to taste. Add the tomato puree and water and bring to a simmer, stirring occasionally. Stir in the sugar erythritol and taste for additional seasoning.

PER SERVING ★ CALORIES: 385 ★ GRAMS OF PROTEIN: 15 ★ GRAMS OF FAT: 31 ★ GRAMS OF CARBOHYDRATE: 12 ★ PERCENT OF PROTEIN: 16% ★ PERCENT OF FAT: 72% ★ PERCENT OF CARBOHYDRATE: 12%

2 Preheat the oven to 425°F.

MAKE THE BISCUITS In a large bowl, whisk together the almond flour, baking powder, sea salt, and pepper. Add the butter and pinch with your fingers until pea-sized pieces form. Add the egg and sour cream and mix until smooth. Refrigerate the mixture for 20 minutes. (To save on prep time, you can prepare the biscuit mixture first and while it refrigerates make the Sloppy Joe mixture.)

Dollop the biscuit mixture (6 dollops) over the top of the Sloppy Joe mixture and bake until the biscuits are golden brown and cooked through, 10 to 12 minutes.

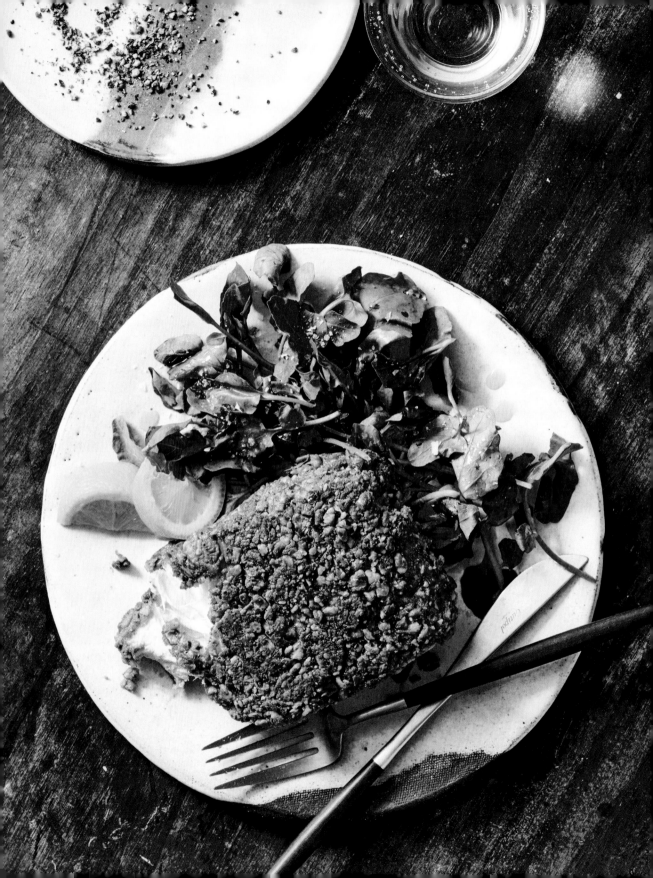

NUT-CRUSTED FISH

PREP TIME: 10 MINUTES ★ COOK TIME: 10 MINUTES ★ SERVINGS: 4

Nuts are a popular addition to dessert recipes, but are equally useful on the savory side of the menu. They play a sensational role in coating fish for a crunchy texture and taste—which is why you'll love this recipe. The first time I tried it, to say I was pleased was an understatement.

½ cup almond flour

1 teaspoon sweet paprika

1 teaspoon lemon-pepper

Pinch of cayenne pepper

Celtic sea salt

3 large eggs, beaten

1 cup of your favorite finely ground nuts

1 tablespoon unsalted grass-fed butter

1 tablespoon extra-virgin olive oil

4 (6-ounce) skinless fish fillets (I tested the recipe with halibut)

1. Set up a dredging station: Place the almond flour, paprika, lemon-pepper, cayenne, and sea salt to taste in a shallow bowl. Place the eggs in a second bowl and the ground nuts in a third.

2. Heat a large nonstick or cast-iron pan over medium-high heat and add the butter and olive oil. Dredge the fish fillets in the seasoned almond flour, shaking off any excess. Dip in the eggs and then coat in the ground nuts. Place in the pan and cook until the fish is cooked through and golden brown on both sides, 2 to 4 minutes per side, depending on the thickness of the fillets. Serve hot.

PER SERVING ★ CALORIES: 344 ★ GRAMS OF PROTEIN: 38 ★ GRAMS OF FAT: 20 ★ GRAMS OF CARBOHYDRATE: 3 ★ PERCENT OF PROTEIN: 44% ★ PERCENT OF FAT: 52% ★ PERCENT OF CARBOHYDRATE: 4%

THE ULTIMATE MEATLOAF

PREP TIME: 15 MINUTES ★ COOK TIME: 1 HOUR 5 MINUTES ★ SERVINGS: 8

Meatloaf is a true comfort food no matter how you make it. If you're new to cooking, meatloaf is something you cannot screw up. It's about the most forgiving recipe you'll ever make. Adding a little more of this or a little less of that usually doesn't make a heck of a difference in the end.

2 tablespoons extra-virgin olive oil

½ small yellow onion, diced

2 cloves garlic, minced

2 pounds ground beef

½ cup crushed Herbed Parmesan Crisps (page 189) or store-bought Parmesan crisps (such as Whisps)

2 large eggs

2 teaspoons coconut aminos

2 tablespoons chopped fresh parsley

2 teaspoons dried oregano

2 teaspoons dried thyme

½ teaspoon dried rosemary

1 teaspoon Celtic sea salt

Freshly ground black pepper

3 tablespoons tomato puree

1. Preheat the oven to 350°F. Line a baking sheet with foil and grease with 1 tablespoon of the olive oil.

2. In a sauté pan, heat the remaining 1 tablespoon olive oil over medium-high heat. Add the onion and garlic and cook until tender but translucent, about 4 minutes. Allow to cool slightly.

3. In a large bowl, combine the sautéed onion and garlic, the beef, crushed crisps, eggs, coconut aminos, parsley, oregano, thyme, rosemary, sea salt, and pepper and mix until combined.

4. Shape the meat mixture into a loaf on the prepared baking sheet and bake for 40 minutes. Remove and spread the tomato puree on top of the meatloaf. Return to the oven and bake until cooked through and a meat thermometer registers 160°F, another 15 to 20 minutes. Allow to rest for 10 minutes before slicing and serving.

PER SERVING ★ CALORIES: 361 ★ GRAMS OF PROTEIN: 22 ★ GRAMS OF FAT: 29 ★ GRAMS OF CARBOHYDRATE: 3 ★ PERCENT OF PROTEIN: 25% ★ PERCENT OF FAT: 72% ★ PERCENT OF CARBOHYDRATE: 3%

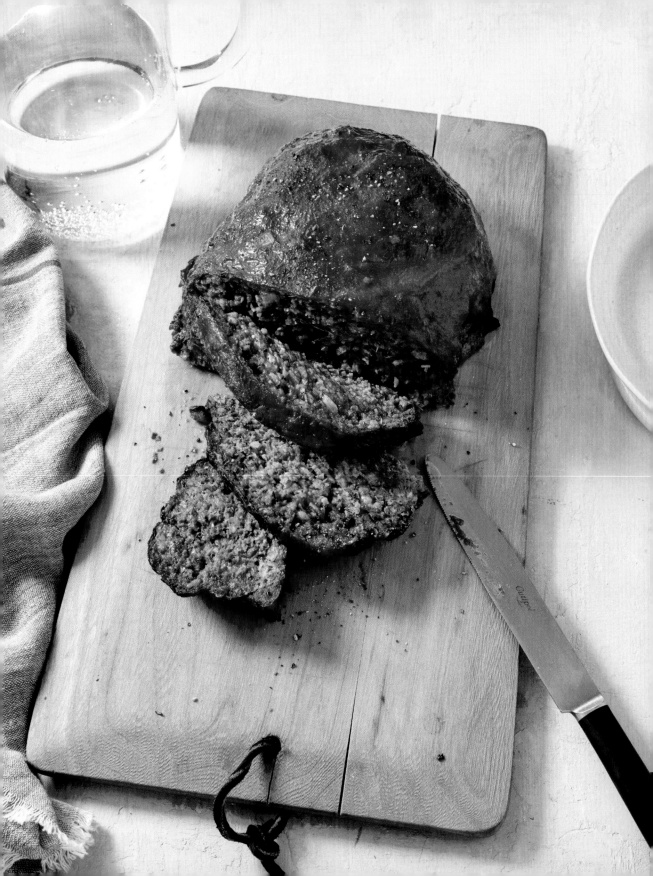

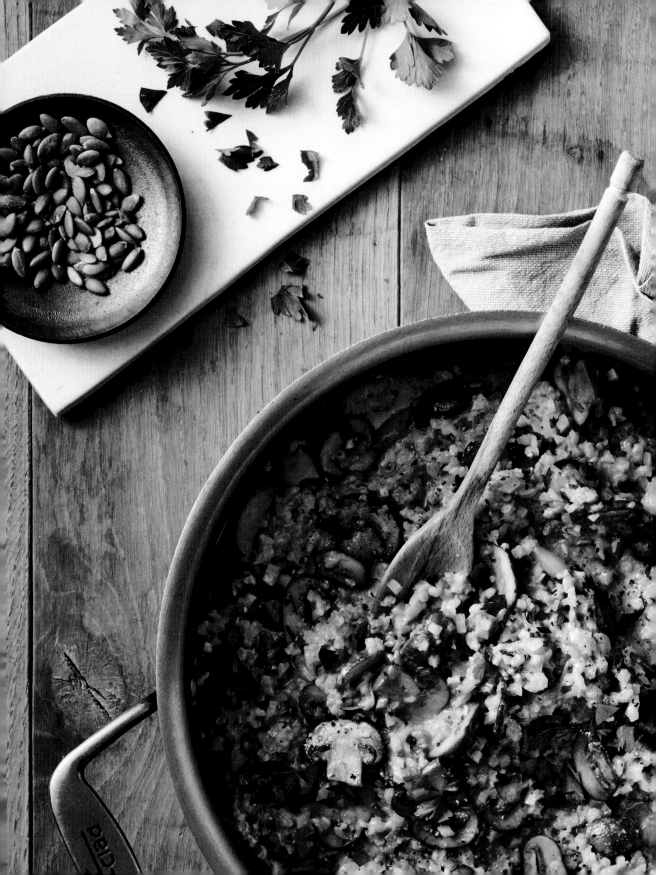

MUSHROOM-CAULIFLOWER RISOTTO WITH PEPITAS

PREP TIME: 10 MINUTES ★ COOK TIME: 15 MINUTES ★ SERVINGS: 4

I can't get enough of low-carb cauliflower! Here I've used it to make "risotto," normally a Northern Italian rice dish cooked in broth until it reaches a creamy consistency. I got to thinking: If cauliflower makes such a great rice substitute, why not turn it into risotto? This lovely vegetarian dish was born.

1 head cauliflower, cut into small florets (or 4 cups store-bought cauliflower rice)

2 tablespoons unsalted grass-fed butter

8 ounces cremini mushrooms, thinly sliced

1 shallot, finely diced

2 cloves garlic, minced

2 teaspoons fresh thyme leaves

Celtic sea salt

Freshly ground black pepper

1 cup chicken stock or vegetable stock

½ cup grated Parmigiano-Reggiano cheese

⅓ cup heavy cream

⅓ cup hulled pumpkin seeds (pepitas), toasted

Chopped fresh parsley

1. In a food processor, pulse the cauliflower florets until they resemble rice. Set aside.

2. In a large sauté pan, heat the butter over medium-high heat. Add the mushrooms and cook until golden brown and almost tender, 6 to 7 minutes. Add the shallot, garlic, and thyme and cook another 2 to 3 minutes, until the shallot is translucent. Season with salt and pepper to taste.

3. Add the cauliflower rice and sauté for 2 to 3 minutes, until the cauliflower is tender. Add the chicken stock and bring to a simmer. Allow the stock to reduce by half, stirring occasionally. Season again with salt and pepper. Remove the pan from the heat and stir in the Parmigiano and cream.

4. Serve sprinkled with the toasted pumpkin seeds and chopped parsley.

PER SERVING ★ CALORIES: 309 ★ GRAMS OF PROTEIN: 15 ★ GRAMS OF FAT: 21 ★ GRAMS OF CARBOHYDRATE: 15 ★ PERCENT OF PROTEIN: 20% ★ PERCENT OF FAT: 60% ★ PERCENT OF CARBOHYDRATE: 20%

SOUPS, STEWS + SALADS

Sticking to a keto diet is easy when "good for you" tastes great, too. That's exactly what I'm serving up in this chapter.

Salads are powerhouses of vegetables and fiber. Soup is one of those foods classified as "low energy dense," meaning that it's low-calorie with high water content. Translation: Soup fills you up without filling you out. As for stews, they're all of the above.

Any of these healthy pleasures can be enjoyed at lunch or dinner. They're examples of how simple and delicious a keto diet can be.

KETO BEEF BONE BROTH

PREP TIME: 10 MINUTES ★ COOK TIME: 17½ HOURS ★ SERVINGS: 6 (1 CUP PER SERVING)

Bone broth is one of the new health foods because of its high mineral and collagen content. This recipe is an important part of my 3-Day Keto Cleanse. It is made by first roasting beef marrow bones and then simmering them for several hours until they break down and release protein and minerals. You can also make bone broth with pork, poultry (chicken or turkey), or fish bones. I add a bunch of veggies to my bone broths for extra nutrition. Also, bone broth makes a great stock for all kinds of soups. You can freeze it for future use.

2½ pounds beef marrow bones

2 tablespoons ghee

1 yellow onion, quartered

2 carrots, peeled and cut into 1-inch pieces

3 stalks celery, cut into 1-inch pieces

1 tablespoon black peppercorns, cracked

Parsley stems (optional)

2 bay leaves (optional)

½ bunch thyme, tied together

2 tablespoons apple cider vinegar

Celtic sea salt

6 tablespoons MCT oil

1. Preheat the oven to 450°F. Line a baking sheet with foil.

2. Arrange the bones on the baking sheet and roast until deep golden brown, 1 hour to 1 hour 30 minutes, flipping the bones halfway through.

3. In a large pot, heat the ghee over medium-high heat. Add the onion, carrots, and celery and cook until softened, about 8 minutes. Add the marrow bones, peppercorns, parsley stems (if using), bay leaves (if using), and thyme. Add water to cover and the vinegar. Bring to a boil, then reduce to a simmer and cook covered for at least 12 and up to 16 hours.

4. Strain the stock (discard the solids) and season with sea salt to taste.

5. For each 1-cup serving of bone broth, stir in 1 tablespoon MCT oil.

PER SERVING ★ CALORIES: 104 ★ GRAMS OF PROTEIN: 0 ★ GRAMS OF FAT: 7 ★ GRAMS OF CARBOHYDRATE: 0 ★ PERCENT OF PROTEIN: 0% ★ PERCENT OF FAT: 100% ★ PERCENT OF CARBOHYDRATE: 0%

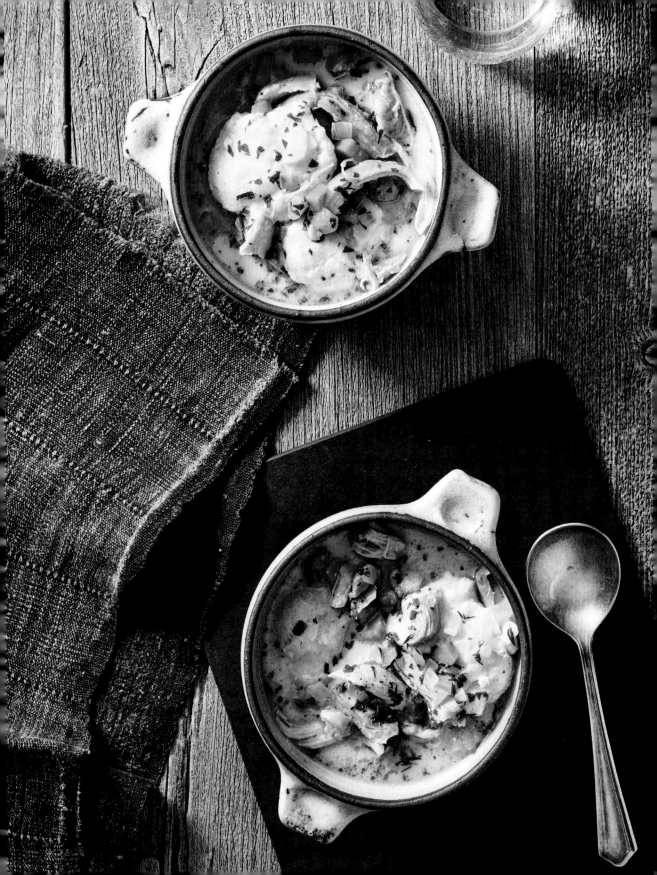

CHICKEN AND DUMPLING SOUP

PREP TIME: 15 MINUTES ★ COOK TIME: 45 MINUTES ★ SERVINGS: 6

Legendary as a soul-warming folk medicine, chicken soup could be the ideal food. I've added yummy dumplings here for an extra measure of comfort. It is theorized that chicken soup has some anti-inflammatory properties. Last winter after coming down with a bad cold, I treated myself to this soup. Within a few days, I no longer had to line my pockets with loads of tissues before leaving home.

CHICKEN SOUP

2 tablespoons extra-virgin olive oil

½ pound boneless, skinless chicken thighs, cut into 1-inch pieces

Celtic sea salt

Freshly ground black pepper

½ yellow onion, diced

1 stalk celery, diced

1 small carrot, diced

2 cloves garlic, minced

2 teaspoons fresh thyme

4 cups chicken stock

2 tablespoons chopped fresh parsley

⅓ cup heavy cream

DUMPLINGS

1 cup shredded low-moisture whole-milk mozzarella cheese

2 tablespoons full-fat cream cheese

¾ cup almond flour

½ teaspoon baking powder

Celtic sea salt

Freshly ground black pepper

1 large egg, beaten

(recipe continues)

1. MAKE THE CHICKEN SOUP: In a large pot or Dutch oven, heat the olive oil over high heat until shimmering. Season the chicken with salt and pepper, add to the pot, and cook until golden brown on all sides and almost cooked through, about 8 minutes total. Remove the chicken to a plate.

2. Add the onion, celery, and carrot to the pot and cook until tender, about 5 minutes. Add the garlic during the last minute of cooking. Add the thyme and season with salt and pepper. Return the chicken to the pot, then add the chicken stock, bring to a boil, and reduce to a simmer. Cook for 25 minutes to meld the flavors and season again with salt and pepper to taste. Stir in the parsley and cream and reduce the heat to the lowest simmer setting.

3. MEANWHILE, MAKE THE DUMPLINGS: Place the mozzarella and cream cheese in a microwave-safe bowl. Microwave at 30-second intervals, stirring after each, until melted and smooth. Add the almond flour and baking powder and season with salt and pepper. Once cooled slightly, add the beaten egg and stir until a dough forms. Remove the dough to a piece of parchment paper and roll into 12 small balls.

4. Drop the dumplings into the simmering soup and cook until lightly puffed, 30 seconds to 1 minute. Do not simmer on a high setting or for too long or the dumplings will fall apart!

PER SERVING ★ CALORIES: 362 ★ GRAMS OF PROTEIN: 20 ★ GRAMS OF FAT: 26 ★ GRAMS OF CARBOHYDRATE: 12 ★ PERCENT OF PROTEIN: 22% ★ PERCENT OF FAT: 65% ★ PERCENT OF CARBOHYDRATE: 13%

BROCCOLI-CHEDDAR SOUP

PREP TIME: 8 MINUTES ★ COOK TIME: 18 MINUTES ★ SERVINGS: 4

When I was a kid, my mom fed me soup when I felt sick. Although she's gone, I still look to soup when I don't feel good. It always makes me feel better. I believe that's because it contains nutrients that help the body recover. Or maybe it reminds me of the love and comfort I got from my mother when she fixed me soup. Either way, soup has always been one of my favorite comfort foods, especially this recipe.

2 cups roughly chopped broccoli

3 tablespoons unsalted grass-fed butter

½ yellow onion, finely chopped

2 cloves garlic, minced

Celtic sea salt

Freshly ground black pepper

3 tablespoons full-fat cream cheese

1¼ cups whole milk

1 cup chicken or vegetable stock

1½ cups shredded sharp cheddar cheese

½ teaspoon xanthan gum

1. Place the broccoli in a microwave-safe bowl. Add 2 tablespoons water and cover with plastic wrap. Poke a hole in the plastic wrap and microwave for 3 to 4 minutes until the broccoli is almost tender. Drain any excess water from the broccoli and set aside.

2. In a large pot, heat the butter over medium-high heat. Add the onion and cook until almost translucent, 5 to 6 minutes. Add the garlic during the last minute and season with salt and pepper to taste. Add the cream cheese and allow to melt. Whisk in the milk and the stock until smooth, bring to a simmer, and cook for 5 minutes, stirring constantly, until thickened. Season again with salt and pepper.

3. Add ¾ cup of the cheddar and whisk until smooth and combined. Add the broccoli and xanthan gum and simmer until slightly thickened, about 1 minute. Serve sprinkled with the remaining cheddar.

PER SERVING ★ CALORIES: 382 ★ GRAMS OF PROTEIN: 17 ★ GRAMS OF FAT: 30 ★ GRAMS OF CARBOHYDRATE: 11 ★ PERCENT OF PROTEIN: 18% ★ PERCENT OF FAT: 71% ★ PERCENT OF CARBOHYDRATE: 11%

LOW-CARB BUTTERNUT SQUASH SOUP

PREP TIME: 15 MINUTES ★ COOK TIME: 35 MINUTES ★ SERVINGS: 4

I love this velvety soup with its sweet, creamy taste, and you will, too. It's the pinnacle of comfort. A special surprise is my addition of health-boosting, spicy ginger. The sage lends a nice herbal flavor.

2 tablespoons coconut oil

½ leek, white and light-green parts only, thinly sliced

2 cloves garlic, minced

1-inch piece fresh ginger, peeled and chopped

⅛ teaspoon freshly grated nutmeg

Celtic sea salt

Freshly ground black pepper

½ head cauliflower, cut into florets (about 2½ cups)

2 cups (½-inch) pieces peeled butternut squash

2 teaspoons fresh thyme leaves

1 teaspoon chopped fresh sage

4 cups vegetable stock or chicken stock

⅔ cup heavy cream

1 tablespoon apple cider vinegar

¼ cup chopped fresh parsley, for garnish

1. In a large pot, heat the coconut oil over medium-high heat. Add the leek and cook until softened, about 6 minutes. Add the garlic, ginger, and nutmeg and cook another minute. Season with salt and pepper to taste.

2. Add the cauliflower and squash and cook until lightly golden, 6 to 7 minutes. Add the thyme and sage and cook an additional minute. Add the stock, bring to a boil, then reduce to a simmer. Cook until the vegetables are tender, about 20 minutes. Season with additional salt and pepper.

3. Transfer the soup to a blender and puree until smooth, then return to the pot. Stir in the cream, season again with salt and pepper, and heat gently to warm through. Stir in the vinegar. Serve garnished with the parsley.

PER SERVING ★ CALORIES: 281 ★ GRAMS OF PROTEIN: 3 ★ GRAMS OF FAT: 21 ★ GRAMS OF CARBOHYDRATE: 20 ★ PERCENT OF PROTEIN: 4% ★ PERCENT OF FAT: 67% ★ PERCENT OF CARBOHYDRATE: 29%

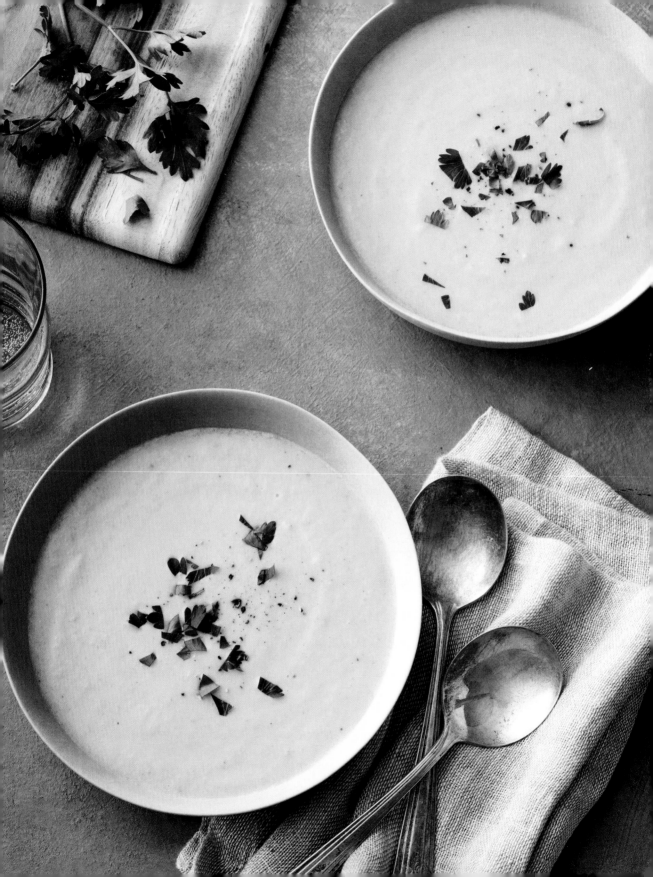

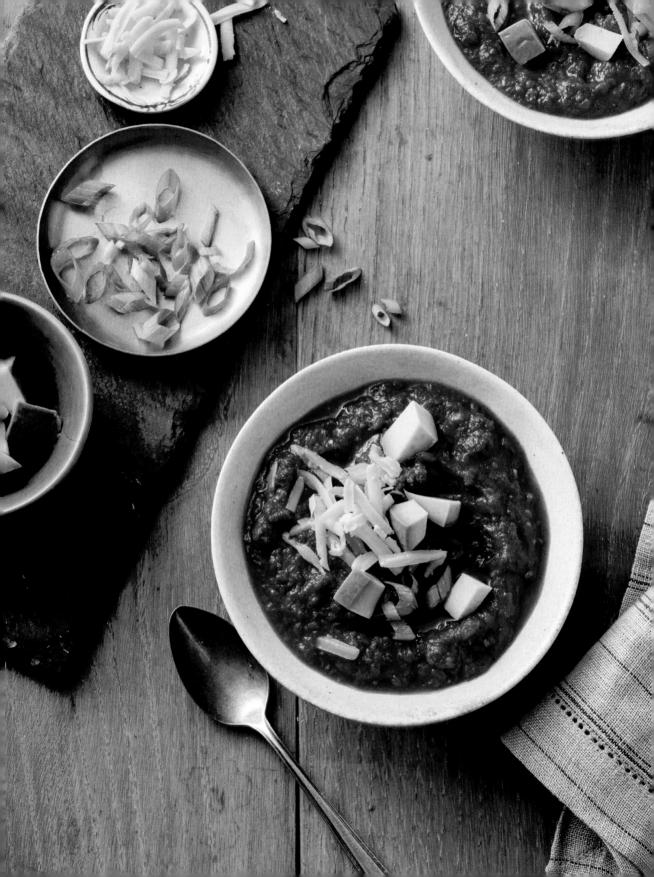

TEXAS-STYLE CHILI

PREP TIME: 10 MINUTES ★ COOK TIME: 35 MINUTES ★ SERVINGS: 6

There are no beans in "real" chili. Just ask a Texan, because that's how they make it in the Lone Star State. I'm fine with that, because Texas chili is definitely a hearty, filling dish to serve up on my Keto Comfort Food Diet.

2 tablespoons extra-virgin olive oil

½ yellow onion, chopped

1 green bell pepper, chopped

4 cloves garlic, minced

Celtic sea salt

Freshly ground black pepper

12 ounces ground beef

3 tablespoons chili powder

1 tablespoon ground cumin

Pinch of cayenne pepper

2 tablespoons coconut aminos

1 (28-ounce) can crushed tomatoes

2 scallions, white and light-green parts only, sliced, for serving

1 avocado, diced, for serving

½ cup shredded sharp cheddar cheese, for serving

1. In a heavy-bottomed pot, heat the olive oil over high heat. Add the onion and bell pepper and cook until almost tender, about 4 minutes. Add the garlic and cook an additional minute. Season with salt and black pepper to taste.

2. Add the ground beef, breaking it up using the back of a wooden spoon. Cook until browned and cooked through, 8 to 10 minutes. Add the chili powder, cumin, cayenne, and coconut aminos, and season with salt and black pepper to taste. Add the crushed tomatoes and stir to combine. Fill half of the tomato can with water, add to the pot, and bring to a simmer. Cook for at least 15 and up to 20 minutes.

3. Serve in bowls topped with the scallions, avocado, and cheddar.

PER SERVING ★ CALORIES: 366 ★ GRAMS OF PROTEIN: 16 ★ GRAMS OF FAT: 25 ★ GRAMS OF CARBOHYDRATE: 20 ★ PERCENT OF PROTEIN: 17% ★ PERCENT OF FAT: 61% ★ PERCENT OF CARBOHYDRATE: 22%

GROUND PORK RAMEN

PREP TIME: 15 MINUTES ★ COOK TIME: 40 MINUTES ★ SERVINGS: 6

If you're a ramen fan, you know it can be addictive and rich in taste. This Japanese dish normally consists of wheat noodles, but I've used no-carb shirataki noodles and flavored it with Asian delights like ginger, mushrooms, scallions, and of course, pork.

This dish is truly delicious, and won't end up on your hips. Make it and enjoy it. I gulped down a generous helping at dinner—and snuck an extra helping when no one was looking.

1 tablespoon toasted sesame oil

2 tablespoons coconut oil

3 cloves garlic, minced

3 scallions, minced

2-inch piece fresh ginger, peeled and grated

8 ounces ground pork

Celtic sea salt

Freshly ground black pepper

8 ounces shiitake mushrooms, stems removed, caps sliced

2 teaspoons chili-garlic sauce

4 cups chicken stock

1 tablespoon coconut aminos

2 teaspoons fish sauce

¼ cup MCT oil

Sriracha (optional)

2 (7-ounce) bags shirataki noodles

½ cup fresh basil, torn

½ cup fresh cilantro, chopped

1 cup bean sprouts

2 limes, cut into wedges, for serving

1. In a large heavy-bottomed pot, heat the sesame oil and coconut oil over medium-high heat. Add the garlic, scallions, and ginger and cook for 2 to 3 minutes, until softened and fragrant. Add the ground pork, breaking it up using the back of a wooden spoon. Cook until browned and cooked through, 7 to 8 minutes. Season with salt and pepper to taste. Add the mushrooms and chili-garlic sauce, and cook until lightly browned, another 6 minutes. Add the chicken stock and bring to a boil. Reduce to a simmer and cook for 20 minutes. Taste, and season again with salt and pepper if needed. Stir in the coconut aminos, fish sauce, MCT oil, and Sriracha to taste (if using).

PER SERVING ★ CALORIES: 297 ★ GRAMS OF PROTEIN: 11 ★ GRAMS OF FAT: 23 ★ GRAMS OF CARBOHYDRATE: 12 ★ PERCENT OF PROTEIN: 15% ★ PERCENT OF FAT: 69% ★ PERCENT OF CARBOHYDRATE: 16%

2. Divide the noodles among 6 bowls (after cooking according to package instructions) and ladle the hot broth over the top. Sprinkle with the basil, cilantro, and bean sprouts. Serve with lime wedges.

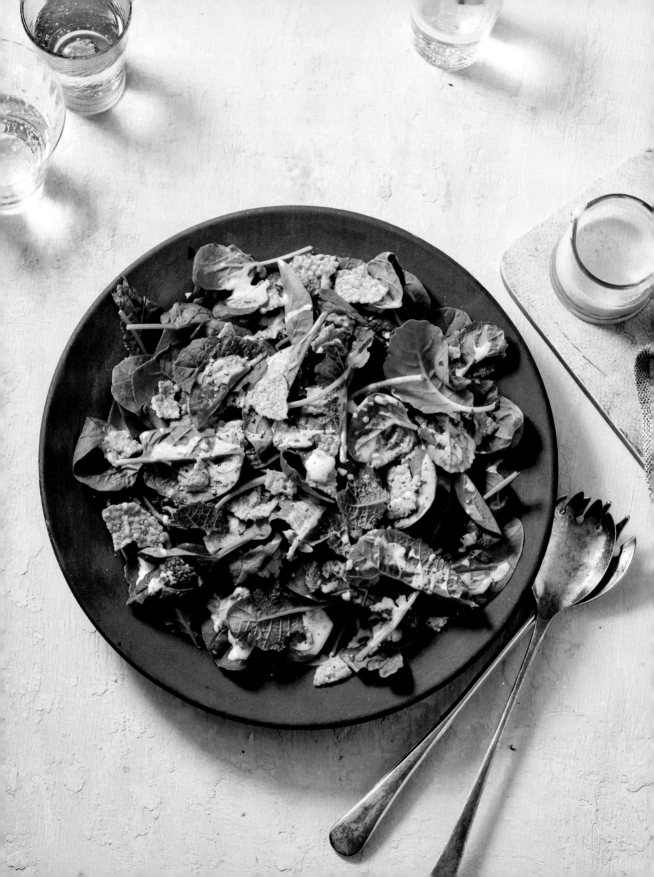

KALE AND SPINACH CAESAR SALAD

PREP TIME: 8 MINUTES ★ SERVINGS: 6

I've changed up the conventional Caesar salad by switching out romaine lettuce for kale and spinach, and I love the makeover. By the way, this popular salad is not named after Julius Caesar as many believe, but after a guy named Caesar Cardini who invented it in 1924 at his restaurant. He was short on salad supplies and had to improvise on the spot. I can attest to the fact that this happens often in the restaurant world. Great recipes are born out of necessity.

CAESAR DRESSING

¾ cup mayonnaise

2 tablespoons fresh lemon juice

2 teaspoons Dijon mustard

1 teaspoon coconut aminos

1 teaspoon anchovy paste

2 cloves garlic, grated

½ cup grated Parmigiano-Reggiano cheese

Celtic sea salt

Freshly ground black pepper

SALAD

1 cup crumbled Herbed Parmesan Crisps (page 189) or store-bought Parmesan crisps (such as Whisps)

3 cups baby kale

3 cups baby spinach

1. MAKE THE CAESAR DRESSING: In a medium bowl, whisk together the mayonnaise, lemon juice, mustard, coconut aminos, anchovy paste, garlic, and Parmigiano. Season with salt and pepper to taste.

2. ASSEMBLE THE SALAD: In a large bowl, toss together the Parmesan crumbles, kale, and spinach. Drizzle ½ cup of the dressing around the rim of the bowl and toss to evenly coat the greens. (Store the remaining dressing in your refrigerator.)

PER SERVING ★ CALORIES: 315 ★ GRAMS OF PROTEIN: 8 ★ GRAMS OF FAT: 29 ★ GRAMS OF CARBOHYDRATE: 5 ★ PERCENT OF PROTEIN: 10% ★ PERCENT OF FAT: 84% ★ PERCENT OF CARBOHYDRATE: 6%

CLASSIC COBB SALAD

PREP TIME: 20 MINUTES ★ COOK TIME: 20 MINUTES, INCLUDING 5 MINUTES TO
PAN-FRY THE BACON ★ SERVINGS: 6

Few salads are as suited to keto cuisine as the Cobb. Blue cheese, bacon, eggs, and avocado are standard ingredients in this dish—and definitely keto-friendly. The Cobb salad was invented at the famed Brown Derby Restaurant in Hollywood and named after its owner, Robert Howard Cobb.

SALAD

3 large eggs

4 cups chopped or torn romaine lettuce

3 cups watercress

6 slices bacon, cooked and chopped

1 avocado, diced

1 large tomato, diced

1 cup crumbled blue cheese

3 scallions, white and light-green parts, thinly sliced

4 fresh chives, chopped

DRESSING

1½ teaspoons Dijon mustard

2 tablespoons red wine vinegar

½ cup extra-virgin olive oil

Celtic sea salt

Freshly ground black pepper

1. **PREPARE THE SALAD:** Set up a bowl of ice and water. Place the eggs in a medium saucepan, add water to cover, and bring to a boil over medium-high heat. Once the water boils, immediately cover the pot and remove from the heat. Let the eggs sit in the hot water for 11 minutes. Transfer the eggs immediately to the ice bath to cool completely. Peel the eggs and chop.

2. In a large bowl, toss together the romaine and watercress. Transfer to a platter or 6 individual plates. Arrange the chopped eggs, bacon, avocado, tomato, and blue cheese in even rows over the salad. Scatter the scallions and chives on top of the salad.

3. **MAKE THE DRESSING:** In a medium bowl, whisk together the mustard and vinegar. While whisking, slowly pour in the olive oil until emulsified. Season with salt and pepper to taste.

4. Drizzle the dressing over the salad and serve.

PER SERVING ★ CALORIES: 384 ★ GRAMS OF PROTEIN: 11 ★ GRAMS OF FAT: 35 ★ GRAMS OF CARBOHYDRATE: 7 ★ PERCENT OF PROTEIN: 11% ★ PERCENT OF FAT: 82% ★ PERCENT OF CARBOHYDRATE: 7%

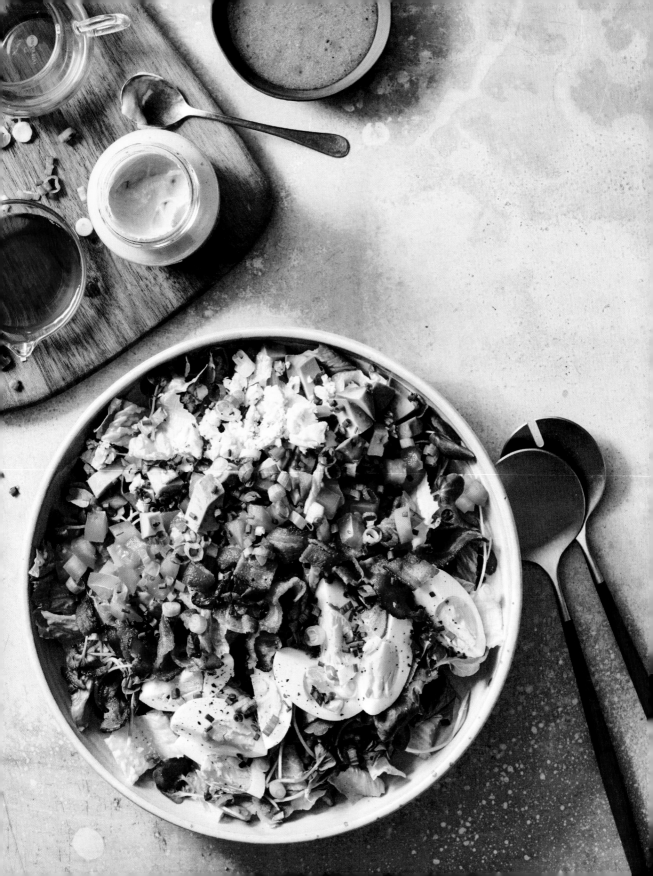

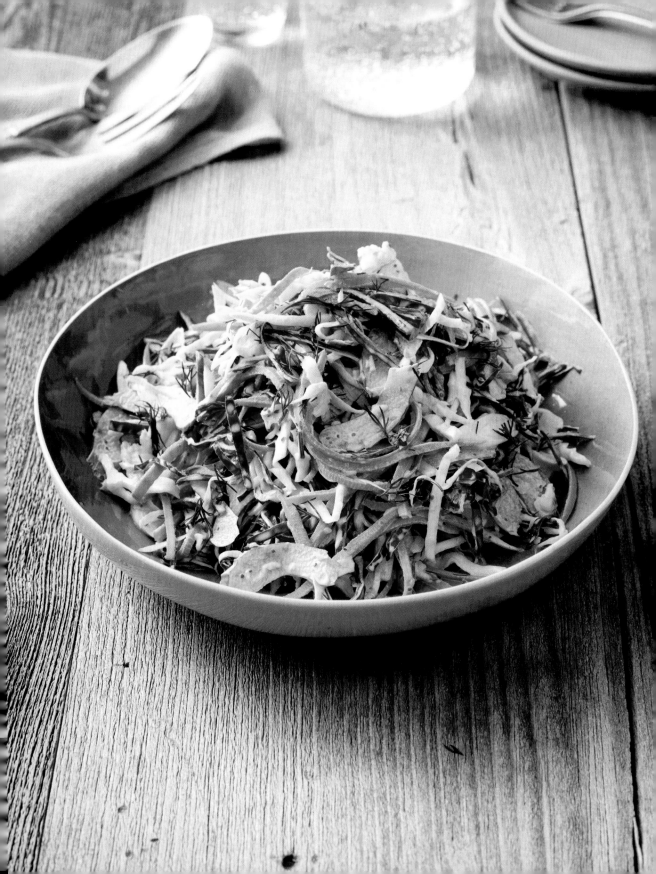

THE CREAMIEST COLESLAW WITH DILL

PREP TIME: 15 MINUTES + 2 HOURS REFRIGERATION ★ SERVINGS: 4

Coleslaw conjures up summer fun, family picnics, outdoor barbecues, and other loving events. It is a perfect keto comfort food salad, with its combination of low-carb veggies and good fats.

½ cup mayonnaise

1 tablespoon apple cider vinegar

1 teaspoon granulated erythritol

1 teaspoon celery seeds

Celtic sea salt

Freshly ground black pepper

2 cups shredded coleslaw mix

3 scallions, white and light-green parts only, thinly sliced on the diagonal

1 stalk celery, thinly sliced on the diagonal

3 tablespoons chopped fresh dill

In a bowl, stir together the mayonnaise, vinegar, erythritol, and celery seeds. Season with salt and pepper to taste. Add the coleslaw mix, scallions, celery, and dill and toss until lightly coated. Cover and refrigerate for 2 hours before serving.

PER SERVING ★ CALORIES: 246 ★ GRAMS OF PROTEIN: 2 ★ GRAMS OF FAT: 22 ★ GRAMS OF CARBOHYDRATE: 10 ★ PERCENT OF PROTEIN: 3% ★ PERCENT OF FAT: 81% ★ PERCENT OF CARBOHYDRATE: 16%

BUFFALO CHICKEN SALAD

PREP TIME: 20 MINUTES ★ COOK TIME: 15 MINUTES ★ SERVINGS: 6

To me, there's nothing more appetizing than Buffalo chicken wings. I decided to "wing" it by creating a salad that would impart all the great flavors of this dish. It features chicken tenders rather than wings, coated in a taste-bud-tantalizing Buffalo sauce. And what is Buffalo chicken without ranch dressing? It's all here—enjoy!

BUFFALO CHICKEN

2 large eggs, beaten

Celtic sea salt

Freshly ground black pepper

2 cups pork rinds, pulsed in a food processor to resemble panko (about ½ cup ground)

½ pound chicken tenders

¼ cup extra-virgin olive oil

3 tablespoons unsalted grass-fed butter, melted

¼ cup hot sauce

CREAMY RANCH DRESSING

¼ cup sour cream

¼ cup mayonnaise

⅓ cup full-fat buttermilk

1 tablespoon fresh lemon juice

1½ teaspoons coconut aminos

½ teaspoon celery salt

1 clove garlic, grated

1 tablespoon chopped fresh chives

1 tablespoon chopped fresh parsley

Celtic sea salt

Freshly ground black pepper

SALAD

8 cups chopped romaine lettuce (1½ to 2 heads)

2 stalks celery, thinly sliced on the diagonal

2 scallions, white and light-green parts only, thinly sliced

½ cup crumbled blue cheese

1. MAKE THE BUFFALO CHICKEN: Set up a dredging station: Place the eggs in a large bowl or shallow baking dish and season with salt and pepper. Place the ground pork rinds in a separate bowl or shallow baking dish. Pat the chicken dry with paper towels and season with salt and pepper. Dip the chicken in the eggs and then in the ground pork rinds, shaking off any excess.

PER SERVING ★ CALORIES: 400 ★ GRAMS OF PROTEIN: 19 ★ GRAMS OF FAT: 33 ★ GRAMS OF CARBOHYDRATE: 8 ★ PERCENT OF PROTEIN: 19% ★ PERCENT OF FAT: 73% ★ PERCENT OF CARBOHYDRATE: 8%

2. In a cast-iron skillet or heavy-bottomed pan, heat the olive oil over medium-high heat until shimmering. Working in batches if necessary, add the chicken tenders to the pan without crowding and cook until golden brown and cooked through, 3 to 4 minutes per side. Remove to a plate lined with paper towels. When cool enough to handle, cut the chicken into 1-inch pieces.

3. In a large bowl, stir together the melted butter and hot sauce. Toss the fried chicken tenders lightly in the butter mixture.

4. MAKE THE CREAMY RANCH DRESSING: In a large bowl, whisk together the sour cream, mayonnaise, buttermilk, lemon juice, coconut aminos, celery salt, garlic, chives, and parsley until smooth. Season with salt and pepper to taste.

5. ASSEMBLE THE SALAD: Divide the romaine among 6 plates and top with celery, scallions, and blue cheese. Serve the creamy ranch dressing on the side. (Alternatively, toss the romaine, celery, scallions, blue cheese, and ranch dressing in a large bowl until evenly coated.) Place the chicken on top of the salad and serve.

VEGGIES + SIDES

Taking up prime real estate in my fridge are nonstarchy vegetables—a mainstay of the Keto Comfort Food Diet. They're easy to "healthy up"—because they're already healthy!

When I don't have time to execute an entire keto comfort food dinner, I throw a steak, pork chop, or piece of chicken or fish on the grill or in the oven and pair it with one of these side dishes. Voilà! I have a fantastic keto comfort food dinner.

ROASTED PORTOBELLO MUSHROOMS

PREP TIME: 5 MINUTES ★ COOK TIME: 20 MINUTES ★ SERVINGS: 4

It's true that I once considered going into the priesthood, but during the past decades, I've been worshipping at the altar of plant-based cuisine (but I'm not giving up lean proteins). One veggie I adore is the portobello mushroom because it's so meaty and flavorful. I've used it in everything, from meatloaf to Sloppy Joes. Here I let it stand on its own, and it does not disappoint.

1 pound portobello or baby bella mushrooms, stems removed, cut into 1-inch pieces

2 tablespoons extra-virgin olive oil

2 cloves garlic, minced

2 teaspoons fresh thyme

Celtic sea salt

Freshly ground black pepper

3 tablespoons red wine vinegar

2 tablespoons ghee, melted

2 tablespoons chopped fresh parsley, for garnish

1. Preheat the oven to 425°F. Line a baking sheet with foil.

2. In a large bowl, toss together the mushrooms, olive oil, garlic, thyme, and salt and pepper to taste until evenly coated.

3. Spread the mushrooms on the baking sheet and roast until golden and tender, 18 to 20 minutes, flipping halfway through. Drizzle the vinegar and ghee over the mushrooms and toss to coat.

4. Serve garnished with the parsley.

PER SERVING ★ CALORIES: 158 ★ GRAMS OF PROTEIN: 3 ★ GRAMS OF FAT: 14 ★ GRAMS OF CARBOHYDRATE: 5 ★ PERCENT OF PROTEIN: 7% ★ PERCENT OF FAT: 80% ★ PERCENT OF CARBOHYDRATE: 13%

CAULIFLOWER MASHED POTATOES

PREP TIME: 5 MINUTES ★ COOK TIME: 30 MINUTES ★ SERVINGS: 4

Mashed cauliflower is the new mashed potato. That may sound clichéd, but it's true. Many restaurants around the country are now offering mashed cauliflower, and I applaud them. The secret to the best mashed cauliflower ever is to roast the cauliflower prior to mashing it. Of course, mixing in keto-friendly cream is a plus, too.

3 cups cauliflower florets

1 tablespoon extra-virgin olive oil, plus more for the baking sheet

Celtic sea salt

Freshly ground black pepper

¾ cup whole-milk plain Greek yogurt

3 tablespoons ghee, melted

¼ cup heavy cream, warmed

1. Preheat the oven to 450°F. Line a baking sheet with foil.

2. Arrange the cauliflower on top of the foil. Drizzle with the 1 tablespoon olive oil and season with salt and pepper to taste. Bring the edges of the foil up to enclose the cauliflower and make a packet.

3. Roast the cauliflower for 20 minutes. Open the foil packet, being careful of the steam, and return to the oven until the cauliflower is tender, another 10 minutes.

4. Transfer the cauliflower to a food processor and add the yogurt, ghee, and cream. Puree until very smooth and season to taste with salt and pepper. Serve hot.

TIP: Try adding your favorite spices, cheeses, or even bacon to this mashed cauliflower—you won't be disappointed!

PER SERVING ★ CALORIES: 217 ★ GRAMS OF PROTEIN: 4 ★ GRAMS OF FAT: 21 ★ GRAMS OF CARBOHYDRATE: 3 ★ PERCENT OF PROTEIN: 7% ★ PERCENT OF FAT: 87% ★ PERCENT OF CARBOHYDRATE: 6%

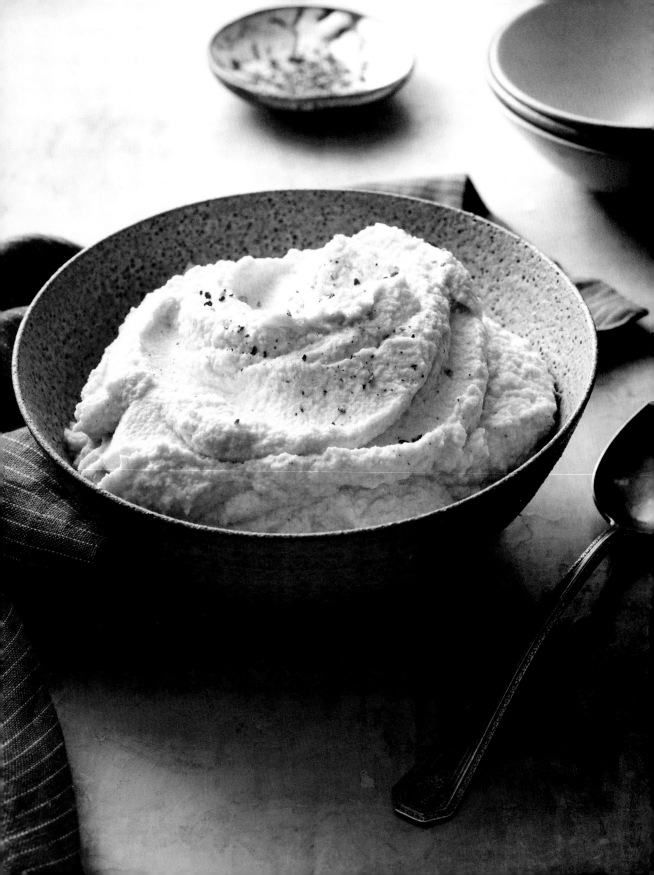

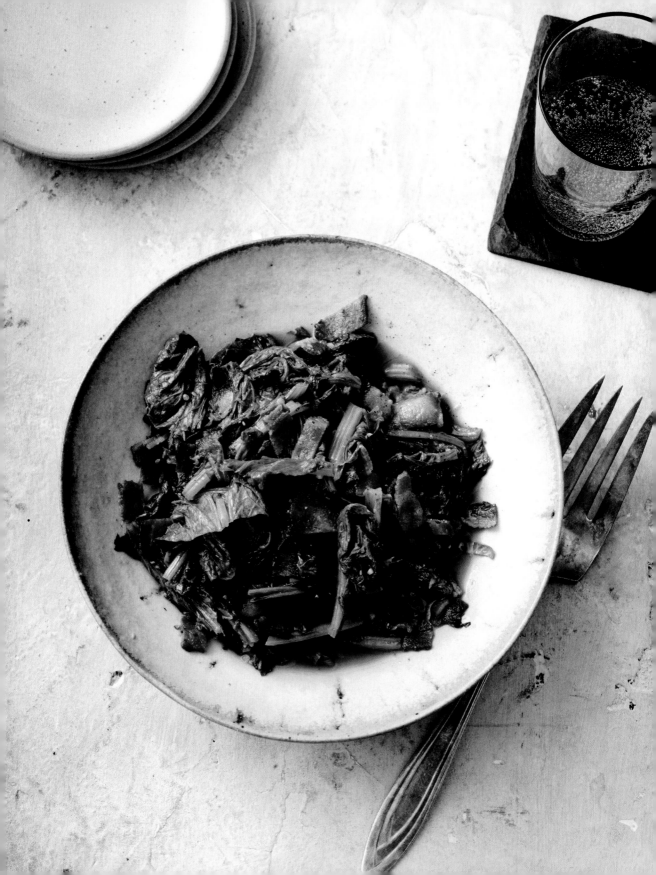

MUSTARD GREENS WITH BACON, GARLIC, AND GINGER

PREP TIME: 10 MINUTES ★ COOK TIME: 20 MINUTES ★ SERVINGS: 4

If you're stuck on spinach but want a change, let me introduce you to mustard greens. Cooked, they impart a rich, earthy flavor that rivals the tastiness of kale, spinach, and other greens. Sauté this tasty leafy green with bacon as this recipe does. That's happiness!

4 slices bacon, cut into ½-inch pieces

2 cloves garlic, minced

1 tablespoon grated peeled fresh ginger

Pinch of red pepper flakes

8 cups mustard greens (1 pound), stemmed and roughly chopped

Celtic sea salt

Freshly ground black pepper

¼ cup chicken stock

1 tablespoon apple cider vinegar

1. Place the bacon in a cold heavy-bottomed sauté pan and heat over medium-high heat. Cook until browned and crispy, at least 7 and up to 9 minutes. With a slotted spoon, transfer the bacon to a plate lined with paper towels.

2. Add the garlic, ginger, and pepper flakes to the bacon fat in the pan and cook for 2 minutes. Add the mustard greens in batches and allow them to wilt. Season to taste with salt and black pepper. Add the chicken stock and continue to cook until tender, another 5 to 6 minutes. Add the vinegar during the last minute of cooking. Serve hot.

PER SERVING ★ CALORIES: 70 ★ GRAMS OF PROTEIN: 6 ★ GRAMS OF FAT: 2 ★ GRAMS OF CARBOHYDRATE: 7 ★ PERCENT OF PROTEIN: 34% ★ PERCENT OF FAT: 26% ★ PERCENT OF CARBOHYDRATE: 40%

"MACARONI" AND CHEESE

PREP TIME: 10 MINUTES ★ COOK TIME: 1 HOUR ★ SERVINGS: 6

Maybe you looked at the title of this recipe and wondered how I'm going to pull off a keto version. Well, it's pretty easy—cauliflower to the rescue again. The mac and cheese everyone buys these days is so full of carbs and preservatives that it should not even be considered. Try this instead. It's totally natural, packed with nutrients, very low-carb, and gluten-free. It's the perfect dish for health-conscious mac and cheese lovers.

2 tablespoons unsalted grass-fed butter, plus 1 tablespoon melted butter for the pan

1 head cauliflower, cut into small florets (3½ to 4 cups)

1 tablespoon extra-virgin olive oil

Celtic sea salt

Freshly ground black pepper

½ yellow onion, roughly chopped

3 cloves garlic, smashed

¼ cup water

½ teaspoon mustard powder

Pinch of cayenne pepper

4 ounces full-fat cream cheese

¾ cup whole milk

1. Preheat the oven to 450°F. Grease an 8 x 8-inch baking dish with the 1 tablespoon melted butter. Line a baking sheet with foil.

2. Arrange the cauliflower on top of the foil. Drizzle with the olive oil and season with salt and black pepper to taste. Bring the edges of the foil up to enclose the cauliflower and make a packet.

3. Roast the cauliflower for 20 minutes. Open the foil packet, being careful of the steam, and return to the oven until the cauliflower is tender, another 15 to 20 minutes. (Leave the oven on.)

4. In a food processor, combine the onion, garlic, and water and pulse until smooth.

PER SERVING ★ CALORIES: 341 ★ GRAMS OF PROTEIN: 15 ★ GRAMS OF FAT: 27 ★ GRAMS OF CARBOHYDRATE: 10 ★ PERCENT OF PROTEIN: 17% ★ PERCENT OF FAT: 71% ★ PERCENT OF CARBOHYDRATE: 12%

1½ cups grated sharp cheddar cheese

1 cup pork rinds, pulsed in a food processor to resemble panko bread crumbs

¼ cup grated Parmigiano-Reggiano cheese

5. In a medium saucepan, heat the 2 tablespoons butter over medium heat. Add the onion and garlic mixture, season with salt and black pepper, and cook for 2 minutes, until the onion begins to soften. Add the mustard powder and cayenne and cook an additional minute. Add the cream cheese and whole milk and allow to melt and come to a simmer. Season with salt and black pepper to taste. Stir in the cheddar until melted and smooth.

6. In a large bowl, toss together the cauliflower and cheese sauce until completely coated. Transfer to the prepared baking dish. Sprinkle the crumbled pork rinds and Parmigiano over the top of the cauliflower and cheese. Bake until golden brown and warmed through, about 10 minutes. Allow to cool for 5 minutes before serving.

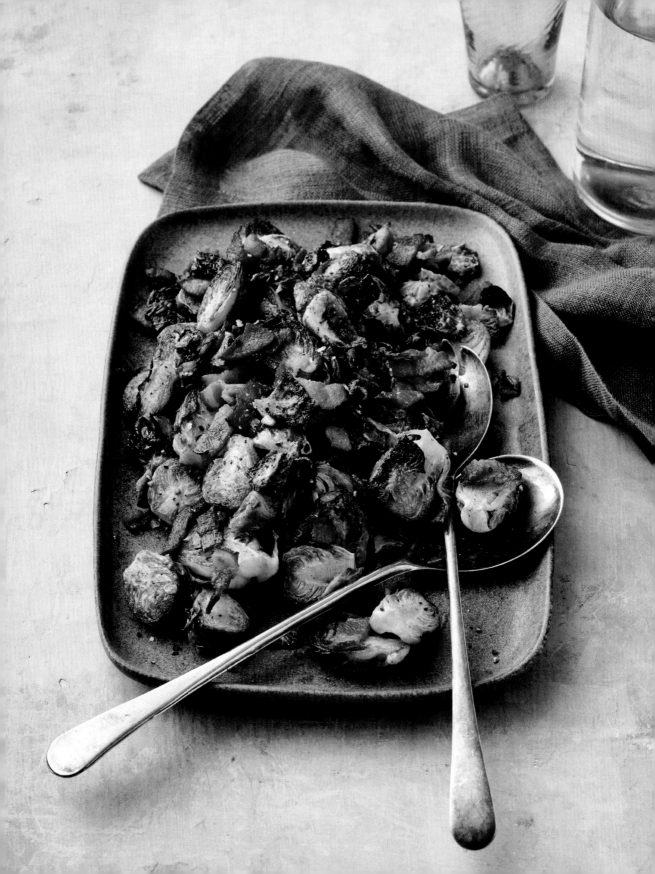

SPICY BACON BRUSSELS SPROUTS

PREP TIME: 5 MINUTES ★ COOK TIME: 20 MINUTES ★ SERVINGS: 4

I've met a lot of people who turn their noses up at Brussels sprouts. I've never understood why. But if you're not in the Brussels sprouts fan club, let me assure you: A little bacon goes a long way to making these babies super delicious.

4 slices bacon, cut into ½-inch pieces

2 tablespoons extra-virgin olive oil

1 pound Brussels sprouts, halved

Celtic sea salt

Freshly ground black pepper

¼ teaspoon liquid stevia

⅛ teaspoon cayenne pepper

1. Place the bacon in a cold cast-iron skillet or heavy-bottomed pan and heat over medium-high heat. Cook until browned and crispy, 7 to 8 minutes. With a slotted spoon, transfer the bacon to a plate lined with paper towels.

2. Add the olive oil to the bacon fat in the pan and heat until shimmering. Add the Brussels sprouts and cook, stirring occasionally, until lightly browned and tender, 10 to 12 minutes. Season with salt and black pepper to taste. Add the liquid stevia, cayenne, and bacon and toss to evenly combine.

PER SERVING ★ CALORIES: 145 ★ GRAMS OF PROTEIN: 6 ★ GRAMS OF FAT: 9 ★ GRAMS OF CARBOHYDRATE: 10 ★ PERCENT OF PROTEIN: 16% ★ PERCENT OF FAT: 56% ★ PERCENT OF CARBOHYDRATE: 28%

PARMESAN HERBED ZUCCHINI FRIES

PREP TIME: 10 MINUTES ★ COOK TIME: 25 MINUTES ★ SERVINGS: 4

Confession time: Who in their weakest moment hasn't fallen prey to the allure of French fries at the drive-through window? So rather than tempt myself, I created this delicious keto-friendly version of fries. Enjoy!

Olive oil or avocado oil cooking spray

½ cup almond flour

¼ cup grated Parmigiano-Reggiano cheese

1 teaspoon Celtic sea salt

½ teaspoon dried oregano

½ teaspoon garlic powder

¼ teaspoon sweet paprika

Pinch of red pepper flakes

2 large eggs, beaten

3 medium zucchini, cut into sticks ¼ to ½ inch thick

3 tablespoons chopped fresh parsley

Low-sugar ketchup (optional), for serving

1. Preheat the oven to 425°F. Line a baking sheet with foil and coat the foil with cooking spray.

2. Set up a dredging station: Stir the almond flour, Parmigiano, sea salt, oregano, garlic powder, paprika, and pepper flakes together in a shallow bowl. Place the beaten eggs in a second shallow bowl.

3. Working in batches, dip the zucchini sticks into the eggs, shaking to remove any excess, and roll them in the herbed cheese mixture to coat. Arrange the coated zucchini sticks on the prepared baking sheet. Bake until golden and crisp, 20 to 25 minutes, turning once halfway.

4. Garnish with the parsley and serve with low-sugar ketchup if desired.

PER SERVING ★ CALORIES: 156 ★ GRAMS OF PROTEIN: 10 ★ GRAMS OF FAT: 10 ★ GRAMS OF CARBOHYDRATE: 6 ★ PERCENT OF PROTEIN: 26% ★ PERCENT OF FAT: 58% ★ PERCENT OF CARBOHYDRATE: 16%

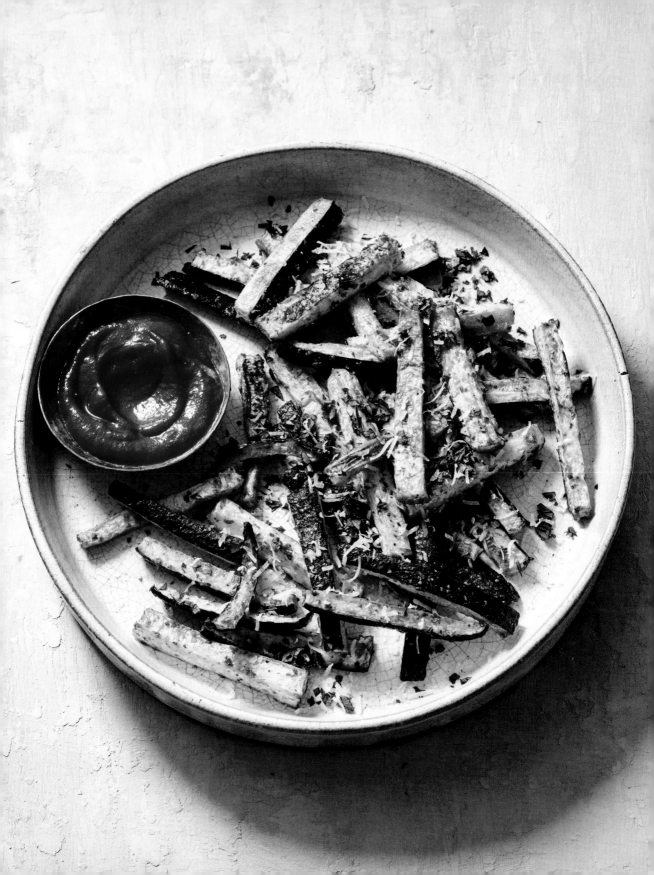

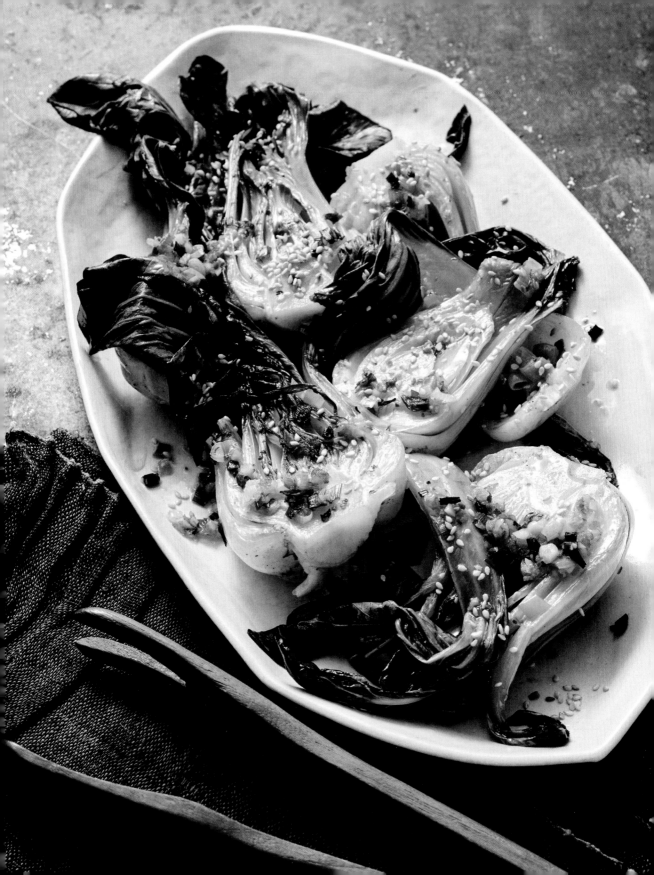

BRAISED BABY BOK CHOY

PREP TIME: 5 MINUTES ★ COOK TIME: 22 MINUTES ★ SERVINGS: 4

Bok choy may not be something you normally have in your veggie bin, but maybe you should! This vegetable has a mild, sweet flavor that lends itself to stir-fries, soups, salads, and everything in between. It's a great way to get a green fix if you ever tire of spinach or kale.

1 tablespoon toasted sesame oil

1 tablespoon coconut oil

2 cloves garlic, minced

2 scallions, finely chopped

1-inch piece fresh ginger, peeled and grated

Celtic sea salt

Freshly ground black pepper

4 heads baby bok choy, halved lengthwise

½ cup chicken stock

2 teaspoons coconut aminos

1¼ tablespoons MCT oil

1 tablespoon sesame seeds, toasted, for garnish

1. In a sauté pan with high sides, heat the sesame oil and coconut oil over medium-high heat. Add the garlic, scallions, and ginger and sauté for at least 2 and up to 3 minutes, until softened. Season with salt and pepper to taste. Add the bok choy, cut-side down, and cook until lightly golden (this may be done in batches), 3 to 4 minutes.

2. Add the chicken stock, scraping up any browned bits on the bottom of the pan, and bring to a simmer. Partially cover the pan and simmer until the bok choy is tender, another 8 to 10 minutes. Stir in the coconut aminos and MCT oil.

3. Serve garnished with the sesame seeds.

PER SERVING ★ CALORIES: 239 ★ GRAMS OF PROTEIN: 2 ★ GRAMS OF FAT: 23 ★ GRAMS OF CARBOHYDRATE: 6 ★ PERCENT OF PROTEIN: 3% ★ PERCENT OF FAT: 87% ★ PERCENT OF CARBOHYDRATE: 10%

SPAGHETTI SQUASH CARBONARA

PREP TIME: 10 MINUTES ★ COOK TIME: 1 HOUR 10 MINUTES ★ SERVINGS: 4

No one loves pasta more than I do. I have been among the roughly one-third of all Americans who eat pasta three or more times a week. Trouble is, we eat too much of it, and pasta in excess can spell trouble for your waistline and your health. One of the best swaps for pasta is spaghetti squash, a large, oblong, yellow squash variety low in carbs. When cooked, the flesh can be flaked with a fork into spaghetti-like strands.

1 spaghetti squash (about 2 pounds), halved lengthwise and seeds scooped out

1 tablespoon extra-virgin olive oil

Celtic sea salt

Freshly ground black pepper

3 slices bacon, chopped

2 tablespoons finely diced yellow onion

3 cloves garlic, minced

⅔ cup whole milk

½ cup grated Parmigiano-Reggiano cheese

2 large egg yolks

1. Preheat the oven to 425°F. Line a baking sheet with foil.

2. Grease the cut sides of the spaghetti squash with the olive oil and season with salt and pepper. Place the squash cut-side down on the foil. Bake until the outer skin is tender when poked with a fork, 40 to 50 minutes. Remove from the oven and allow to cool for 10 minutes.

3. Meanwhile, place the bacon in a skillet and place over medium-high heat. Cook until browned and crisp, 6 to 7 minutes. With a slotted spoon, transfer the bacon to a plate lined with paper towels.

4. Add the onion and garlic to the bacon fat in the pan and cook for 4 minutes. Season with salt and pepper to taste. Remove the pan from the heat. Add the milk and Parmigiano and whisk to combine. Add the egg yolks and whisk until the sauce is thickened (the residual heat from the pan is enough to cook the yolks and thicken the sauce). Season again with salt and pepper.

PER SERVING ★ CALORIES: 233 ★ GRAMS OF PROTEIN: 10 ★ GRAMS OF FAT: 13 ★ GRAMS OF CARBOHYDRATE: 19 ★ PERCENT OF PROTEIN: 17% ★ PERCENT OF FAT: 50% ★ PERCENT OF CARBOHYDRATE: 33%

5. Using a fork, pull the strands of spaghetti squash into a large bowl. Pour the hot cream sauce over the top and toss to coat, adding the bacon. Serve on a platter or in the skin of the squash.

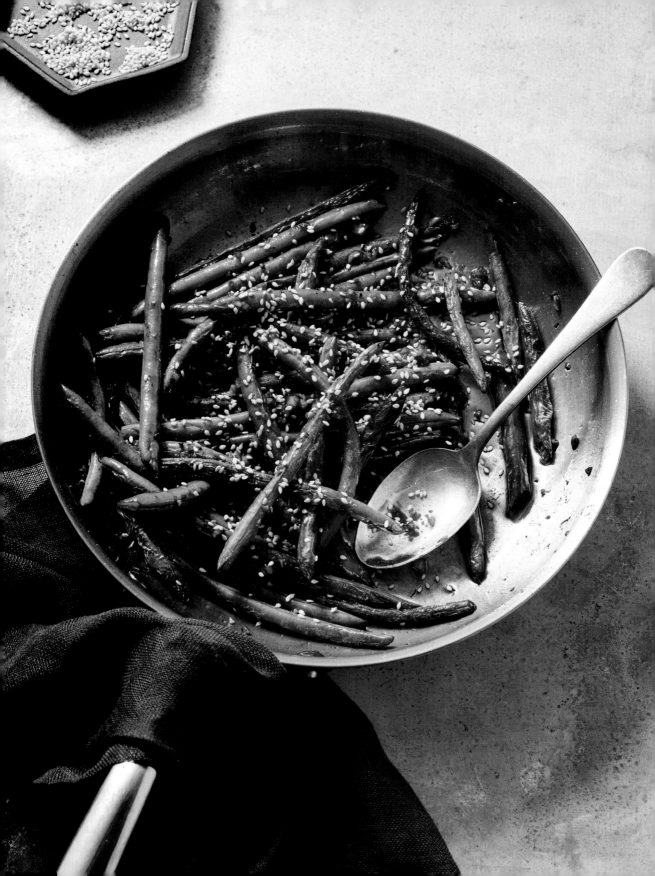

GREEN BEANS IN GARLIC SAUCE

PREP TIME: 5 MINUTES ★ COOK TIME: 10 MINUTES ★ SERVINGS: 4

Green beans are not boring—especially when cooked to crisp-tenderness with keto-friendly oils, garlic, and other spices. You'll love this bold-flavored side dish.

1 tablespoon coconut oil

1 tablespoon toasted sesame oil

1½ pounds green beans, trimmed

4 cloves garlic, minced

1-inch piece fresh ginger, peeled and grated

Pinch of red pepper flakes (optional)

Celtic sea salt

Freshly ground black pepper

2 tablespoons coconut aminos

¼ cup MCT oil

1 tablespoon sesame seeds, toasted, for garnish

1. In a large heavy-bottomed skillet, heat the coconut oil and sesame oil over high heat. Add the green beans and cook until charred and tender, 8 to 10 minutes. Add the garlic and ginger during the last minute of cooking. Season with pepper flakes (if using) and salt and black pepper to taste.

2. Pour the coconut aminos and MCT oil over the green beans and toss to coat until warmed through and slightly reduced.

3. Serve garnished with the sesame seeds.

PER SERVING ★ CALORIES: 287 ★ GRAMS OF PROTEIN: 4 ★ GRAMS OF FAT: 23 ★ GRAMS OF CARBOHYDRATE: 16 ★ PERCENT OF PROTEIN: 6% ★ PERCENT OF FAT: 72% ★ PERCENT OF CARBOHYDRATE: 22%

CREATED SPINACH

PREP TIME: 5 MINUTES ★ COOK TIME: 10 MINUTES ★ SERVINGS: 4

Here's a traditional comfort dish that your mom probably served at family dinners. I bet you never thought you'd get to eat it again to control your weight! Welcome back, creamed spinach!

2 tablespoons unsalted grass-fed butter

½ yellow onion, chopped

2 cloves garlic, minced

Celtic sea salt

Freshly ground black pepper

4 ounces full-fat cream cheese, cut into cubes

½ cup heavy cream

1 (10-ounce) package frozen spinach, thawed and squeezed of excess liquid

⅛ teaspoon freshly grated nutmeg

In a medium saucepan, heat the butter over medium heat. Add the onion and cook until translucent, about 5 minutes. Add the garlic and cook an additional minute. Season with salt and pepper to taste. Add the cream cheese and stir until melted. Add the cream and bring to a simmer. Add the spinach and nutmeg, season with salt and pepper to taste, and stir to combine. Serve hot.

PER SERVING ★ CALORIES: 274 ★ GRAMS OF PROTEIN: 4 ★ GRAMS OF FAT: 26 ★ GRAMS OF CARBOHYDRATE: 6 ★ PERCENT OF PROTEIN: 6% ★ PERCENT OF FAT: 85% ★ PERCENT OF CARBOHYDRATE: 9%

DESSERTS + TREATS

Sugar is synonymous with dessert, right? A long time ago, sugar used to be okay because it was fat-free. But now we know better—that a high-sugar diet can cause heart disease, obesity, diabetes, and other adverse health conditions.

With keto dieting, sugar is out—a benefit of ketogenic nutrition and why it is one of the healthiest diets around.

Because I love desserts—and I bet you do, too—I had to rework a lot of popular recipes to meet my keto comfort food requirements. They had to taste sugary, but without the sugar. A huge challenge—but I met it! The results have been amazing.

Now, dessert is back on the table.

CHOCOLATE AVOCADO MOUSSE

PREP TIME: 10 MINUTES ★ SERVINGS: 4

I love chocolate. Luscious, delicious, erotic, simply heavenly chocolate. I believe chocolate is the antidote for depression and bad moods. Everyone gets happy when they eat chocolate.

But here's the catch: If you're trying to lose or control your weight, chocolate can be one of the first things you crave a few days into a diet, especially if it's laced with sugar. And if you're anything like me, it's hard to work a favorite food like chocolate into your diet without overindulging. So I figured out a way to keto-ize one of my favorite chocolate desserts—chocolate mousse, using the creamy avocado as its base. This healthy fruit creates a mousse that is far better than any you've ever tasted.

1 avocado, halved and pitted

½ cup unsweetened cocoa powder, sifted

1 teaspoon vanilla extract

½ cup confectioners' erythritol

½ cup heavy cream, chilled

1. Scoop the avocado into a food processor and pulse until very smooth. Transfer to a large bowl and stir in the cocoa powder, vanilla, and erythritol until smooth.

2. In a bowl, with an electric mixer, whip the cream to stiff peaks. Gently fold the whipped cream into the avocado mixture. Serve immediately or refrigerate until ready to serve.

PER SERVING ★ CALORIES: 218 ★ GRAMS OF PROTEIN: 3 ★ GRAMS OF FAT: 18 ★ GRAMS OF CARBOHYDRATE: 11 ★ PERCENT OF PROTEIN: 6% ★ PERCENT OF FAT: 74% ★ PERCENT OF CARBOHYDRATE: 20%

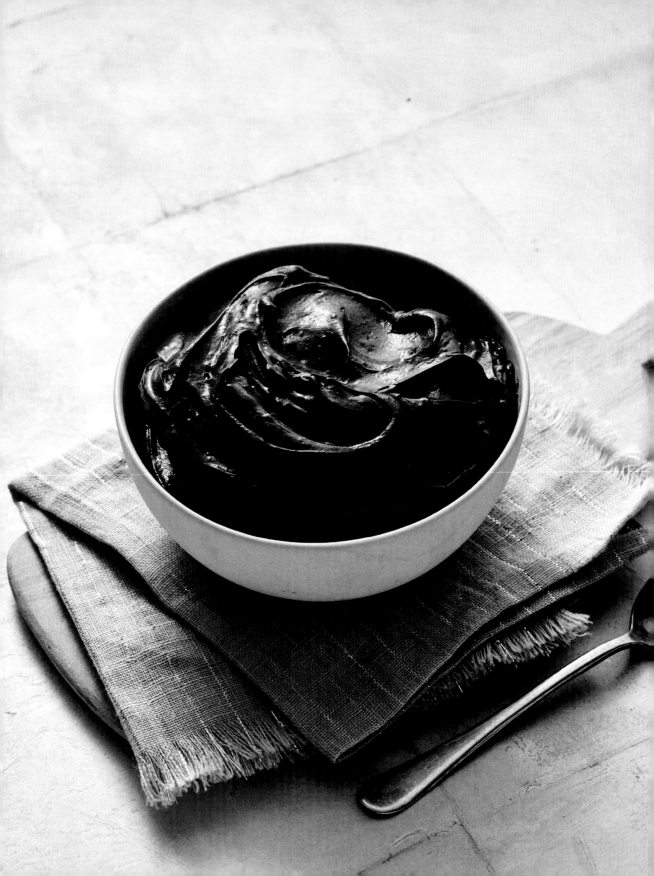

DOUBLE-CHOCOLATE TAHINI BROWNIES

PREP TIME: 15 MINUTES ★ COOK TIME: 22 MINUTES ★ SERVINGS: 8

Ahhhh—brownies! Would you like to bite into a moist, fudge-like brownie now? Here's a recipe you can whip up quickly—one that everyone in your family will love.

½ cup almond flour

2 tablespoons unsweetened cocoa powder

½ teaspoon Celtic sea salt

¾ cup stevia-sweetened dark chocolate baking chips (such as Lily's)

5 tablespoons unsalted grass-fed butter

⅓ cup tahini

2 large eggs

1 teaspoon vanilla extract

1 tablespoon brewed coffee, cooled

¼ cup granulated erythritol

¼ cup brown sugar erythritol

Confectioners' erythritol (optional), for dusting

1. Preheat the oven to 350°F. Line an 8 x 8-inch metal baking dish with parchment paper up two sides.

2. In a bowl, whisk together the almond flour, cocoa powder, and sea salt.

3. Place the chocolate chips and butter in a microwave-safe bowl. Microwave in 30-second intervals, stirring after each, until melted and smooth. Stir the tahini, eggs, vanilla, coffee, granulated erythritol, and brown sugar erythritol into the chocolate mixture. Stir in the almond flour mixture.

4. Scrape the batter into the prepared pan. Bake until an inserted toothpick comes out clean, 18 to 20 minutes. Cool in the pan on a wire rack for 10 minutes.

5. Remove from the pan and cut into 8 brownies. If desired, dust with confectioners' erythritol.

PER SERVING ★ CALORIES: 303 ★ GRAMS OF PROTEIN: 7 ★ GRAMS OF FAT: 23 ★ GRAMS OF CARBOHYDRATE: 17 ★ PERCENT OF PROTEIN: 9% ★ PERCENT OF FAT: 68% ★ PERCENT OF CARBOHYDRATE: 23%

RICOTTA CHEESECAKE WITH STRAWBERRY SAUCE

PREP TIME: 20 MINUTES + 4 HOURS REFRIGERATION TIME ★ COOK TIME: 1 HOUR 20 MINUTES ★ SERVINGS: 8

Who eats cheesecake on a keto diet? You do—with this lovely ricotta cheesecake. It is sugar-free but otherwise doesn't differ from traditional cheesecakes, because with keto cuisine you get to use whole milk and other full-fat products. In fact, it is even richer in taste than most ricotta cheesecakes.

CRUST

¾ cup almond flour

2 tablespoons unsalted grass-fed butter, melted

1 tablespoon granulated erythritol

FILLING

12 ounces full-fat cream cheese, at room temperature

1¼ cups whole-milk ricotta cheese

¼ cup granulated erythritol

1 teaspoon vanilla extract

3 large eggs

1 tablespoon unsalted grass-fed butter, melted

STRAWBERRY SAUCE

½ cup hulled and roughly chopped strawberries

2 tablespoons fresh lemon juice

2 tablespoons water

1 tablespoon granulated erythritol

1. Preheat the oven to 350°F. Cover the outside of an 8-inch springform pan with foil.

2. MAKE THE CRUST: In a food processor, pulse together the almond flour, melted butter, and erythritol until combined. Press the mixture into the bottom of the springform pan and bake until golden brown, 12 to 14 minutes. Allow to cool completely. (Leave the oven on.)

(recipe continues)

3. MAKE THE FILLING: In a stand mixer fitted with the paddle attachment, beat the cream cheese and ricotta until smooth. Add the erythritol and vanilla and mix until combined. Add the eggs and mix until just incorporated, being careful not to overmix.

4. Grease the sides of the springform pan with the melted butter. Pour the filling into the crust. Place the springform pan in a roasting pan and fill the roasting pan with warm water to create a water bath that comes halfway up the sides of the springform pan. Bake until the center of the cheesecake lightly jiggles, 50 minutes to 1 hour. Remove from the water bath, cool to room temperature, then refrigerate for at least 4 hours before serving.

5. MAKE THE STRAWBERRY SAUCE: In a food processor, pulse together the strawberries, lemon juice, water, and erythritol, keeping the strawberries chunky. Transfer to a small saucepan and simmer until slightly thickened, about 5 minutes. Allow to cool.

6. Remove the sides of the springform pan and spoon the strawberry sauce on top.

PER SERVING ★ CALORIES: 351 ★ GRAMS OF PROTEIN: 12 ★ GRAMS OF FAT: 31 ★ GRAMS OF CARBOHYDRATE: 6 ★ PERCENT OF PROTEIN: 14% ★ PERCENT OF FAT: 79% ★ PERCENT OF CARBOHYDRATE: 7%

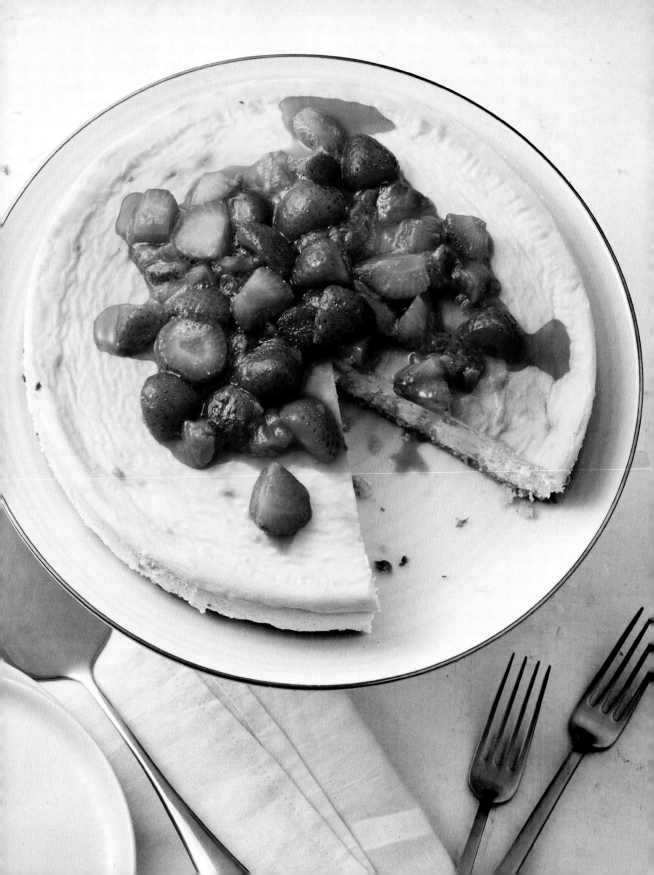

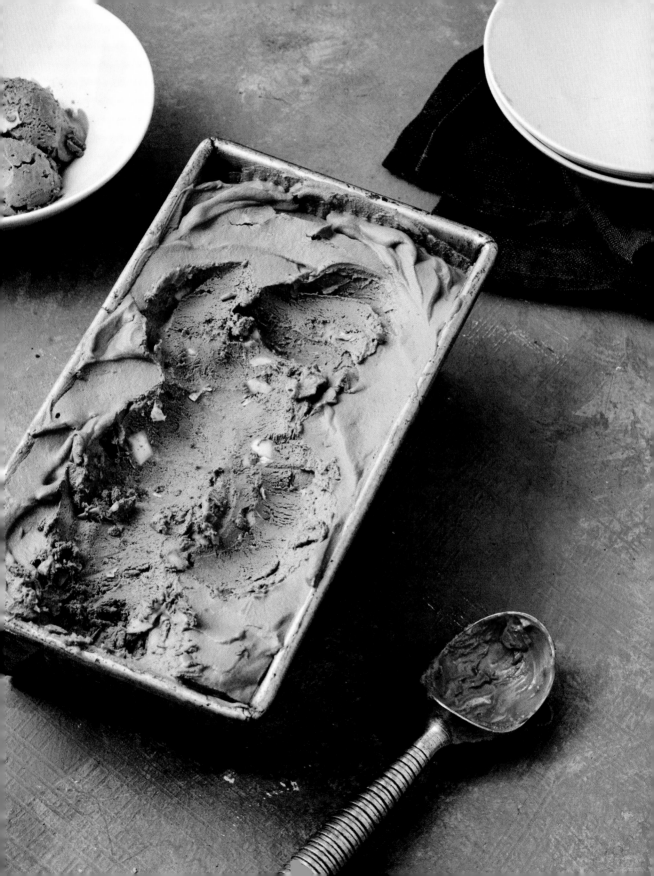

CHOCOLATE COCONUT MACADAMIA ICE CREAM

PREP TIME: 10 MINUTES + 4 HOURS FREEZING ★ COOK TIME: 5 MINUTES ★ SERVINGS: 16

I've been creating healthy versions of ice cream since 2008 because this perennial treat is so important for satisfying a dieter's needs. Developing an ice cream that helps you lose weight is a challenge. I've been known to rework an ice cream recipe twenty or more times before I feel it's right. So I'm proud to present this yummy frozen confection to support you while following my Keto Comfort Food Diet.

½ (14-ounce) can full-fat unsweetened coconut milk

⅓ cup confectioners' erythritol

1 teaspoon vanilla extract

⅓ cup unsweetened cocoa powder

1 tablespoon coconut extract

¼ teaspoon Celtic sea salt

2 cups heavy cream

½ cup unsweetened coconut flakes, toasted

½ cup toasted and chopped macadamia nuts

1. Line a 9 x 5-inch loaf pan with plastic wrap.

2. In a small saucepan, heat the coconut milk. Add the erythritol and whisk until dissolved. Remove from the heat and add the vanilla, cocoa powder, coconut extract, and sea salt. Let the mixture cool completely. Once it is cooled, transfer the mixture into a medium mixing bowl.

3. In a bowl, with an electric mixer, beat the cream to medium peaks. Gently fold the whipped cream into the coconut milk mixture. Add the coconut flakes and macadamia nuts.

4. Scrape the mixture into the prepared loaf pan to freeze for at least 4 hours or until hardened. If the ice cream is very hard, let it sit at room temperature for 30 minutes before serving.

PER SERVING ★ CALORIES: 173 ★ GRAMS OF PROTEIN: 1 ★ GRAMS OF FAT: 17 ★ GRAMS OF CARBOHYDRATE: 4 ★ PERCENT OF PROTEIN: 2% ★ PERCENT OF FAT: 89% ★ PERCENT OF CARBOHYDRATE: 9%

CHOCOLATE PEANUT BUTTER COOKIES

PREP TIME: 10 MINUTES ★ COOK TIME: 10 MINUTES ★ SERVINGS: 12 (2 COOKIES PER SERVING)

When I crave cookies, my scale gets really nervous. That's because in the past I've been known to put on pounds by overindulging in a cookie or two or four. Well, here's a cookie I've put on my Keto Comfort Food Diet by downsizing the carbs and sugar.

¾ cup creamy unsweetened natural peanut butter

1 large egg

1 teaspoon vanilla extract

¼ cup unsweetened cocoa powder

½ cup almond flour

½ teaspoon baking soda

½ cup confectioners' erythritol

1. Preheat the oven to 375°F. Line a baking sheet with parchment paper.

2. In a large bowl, mix together the peanut butter, egg, vanilla, cocoa powder, almond flour, baking soda, and erythritol until smooth.

3. Scoop the dough into 24 (1-inch) balls and flatten with a fork on the prepared baking sheet. Bake until set, 8 to 10 minutes. Let cool completely on the baking sheet. Store in an airtight container for 3 to 4 days.

PER SERVING ★ CALORIES: 143 ★ GRAMS OF PROTEIN: 6 ★ GRAMS OF FAT: 11 ★ GRAMS OF CARBOHYDRATE: 5 ★ PERCENT OF PROTEIN: 17% ★ PERCENT OF FAT: 69% ★ PERCENT OF CARBOHYDRATE: 14%

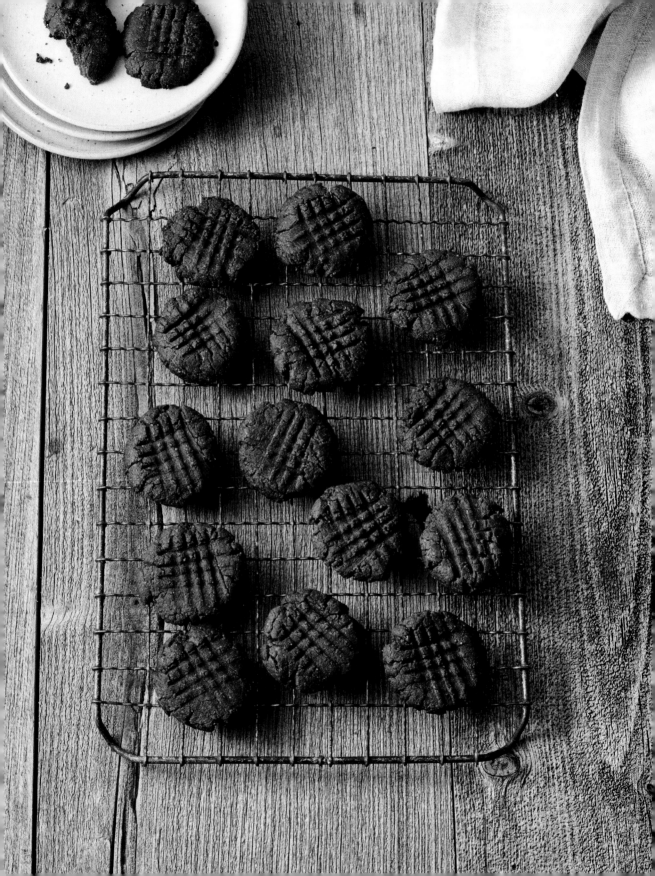

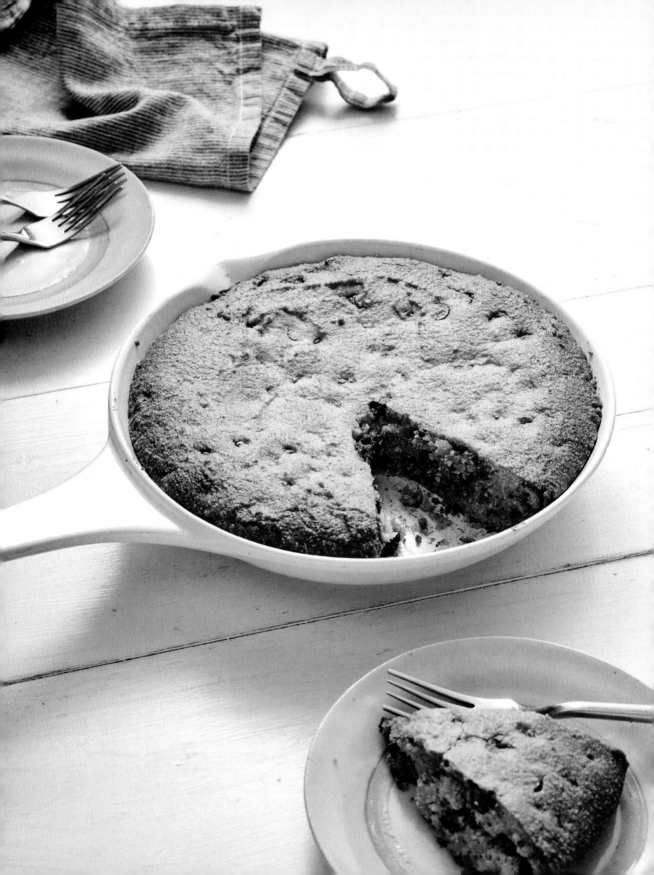

CHOCOLATE CHIP SKILLET COOKIE

PREP TIME: 10 MINUTES ★ COOK TIME: 25 MINUTES ★ SERVINGS: 12

What could be a more comforting sweet treat than a large cookie—
like the ones you see at the mall? Here it is . . . my version of those
iconic cookies craved by cookie lovers everywhere. And yes, you
can eat it and stay in fat-burning ketosis!

1 stick (4 ounces) unsalted
grass-fed butter, at room
temperature, + 1 tablespoon
for the skillet

¼ cup brown sugar erythritol

¼ cup granulated erythritol

2 large eggs

1 teaspoon vanilla extract

½ teaspoon Celtic sea salt

½ teaspoon baking soda

1½ cups almond flour

1 cup stevia-sweetened
dark chocolate baking chips
(such as Lily's)

1. Preheat the oven to 350°F. Grease a 10-inch cast-iron
skillet with the 1 tablespoon butter.

2. In a bowl, with an electric mixer, beat the butter, brown
sugar erythritol, and granulated erythritol until light and
fluffy. Add the eggs, one at a time, beating well after each
addition. Add the vanilla and salt and mix to combine.

3. Add the baking soda and almond flour and mix until
just incorporated. Add the chocolate chips and stir to
combine using a rubber spatula.

4. Pat the cookie dough into the skillet and bake until
golden brown and the middle is almost set, about
25 minutes. Let cool for 10 minutes, cut into wedges,
and serve.

PER SERVING ★ CALORIES: 262 ★ GRAMS OF PROTEIN: 5 ★ GRAMS OF FAT: 22 ★ GRAMS OF CARBOHYDRATE: 11 ★
PERCENT OF PROTEIN: 8% ★ PERCENT OF FAT: 75% ★ PERCENT OF CARBOHYDRATE: 17%

FLOURLESS CHOCOLATE CAKE WITH ALMOND-COCONUT CREAM

PREP TIME: 10 MINUTES ★ COOK TIME: 27 MINUTES ★ SERVINGS: 8

You haven't savored chocolate cake until you've tasted one made without flour. It is simply divine—pure fudgy moistness passing between your lips. I'd much rather go flourless than anything else. Plus, there's absolutely no sugar in this luscious, buttery cake.

Butter and cocoa powder, for the pan

FLOURLESS CHOCOLATE CAKE

1 cup stevia-sweetened semisweet chocolate baking chips (such as Lily's)

1 stick (4 ounces) unsalted grass-fed butter

⅔ cup granulated erythritol

½ teaspoon Celtic sea salt

1 teaspoon vanilla extract

1 tablespoon brewed coffee, cooled

3 large eggs

⅓ cup unsweetened cocoa powder

1. Preheat the oven to 375°F. Grease an 8-inch springform pan with butter and dust with cocoa powder.

2. MAKE THE FLOURLESS CHOCOLATE CAKE: Combine the chocolate chips and butter in a microwave-safe bowl. Microwave in 30-second intervals, stirring after each, until melted and smooth. Stir in the granulated erythritol, salt, vanilla, and coffee to combine. Whisk in the eggs to combine. Add the cocoa powder and fold until just combined.

3. Scrape the batter into the prepared springform pan and bake until the top has formed a thin crust and the center jiggles slightly, about 25 minutes. Remove to a wire rack to cool for 10 minutes.

4. MEANWHILE, MAKE THE ALMOND-COCONUT CREAM: In a bowl, with an electric mixer, whisk together the coconut cream, almond extract, confectioners' erythritol, and cream until soft peaks form. Keep refrigerated until ready to serve.

PER SERVING ★ CALORIES: 292 ★ GRAMS OF PROTEIN: 4 ★ GRAMS OF FAT: 24 ★ GRAMS OF CARBOHYDRATE: 15 ★ PERCENT OF PROTEIN: 6% ★ PERCENT OF FAT: 74% ★ PERCENT OF CARBOHYDRATE: 20%

ALMOND-COCONUT CREAM

¼ cup unsweetened coconut cream

1 teaspoon almond extract

2 tablespoons confectioners' erythritol

2 tablespoons heavy cream

5. Run an offset spatula or a butter knife around the edge of the cake and release the outer ring of the pan. Cut into wedges and serve with a dollop of the almond-coconut cream.

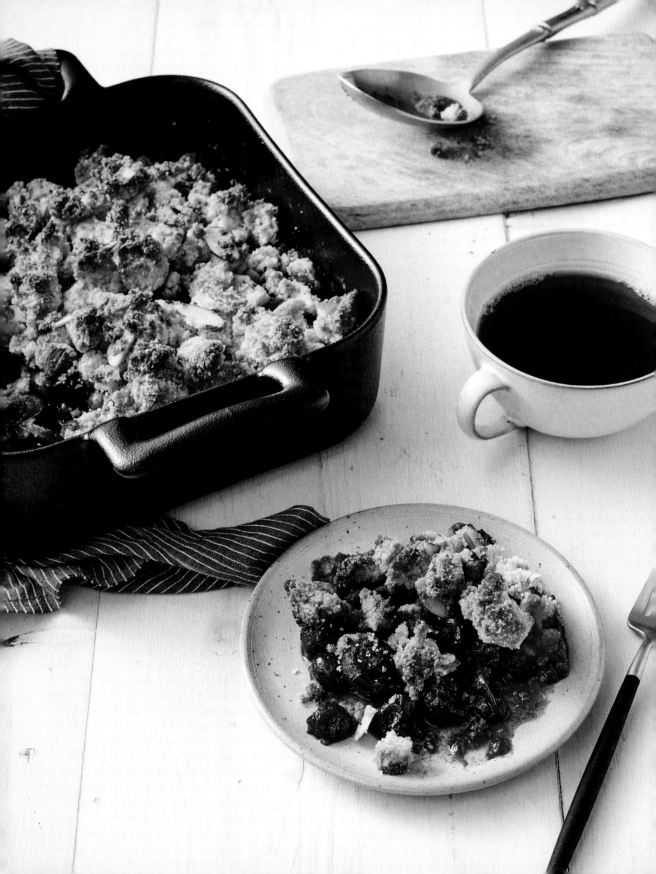

CRANBERRY CHERRY ALMOND CRUMBLE

PREP TIME: 10 MINUTES ★ COOK TIME: 25 MINUTES ★ SERVINGS: 8

A popular finish to dinner is this fruity treat—a takeoff on cherry cobbler but without all the carbs, sugar, and other fattening stuff. It's super easy to make and leftovers refrigerate well. The cranberries add an unexpected zest to this mouthwatering dessert.

Vegetable oil cooking spray

CRANBERRY-CHERRY FILLING

1½ cups frozen pitted sweet dark cherries (you can bake them frozen)

1½ cups frozen cranberries

2 tablespoons granulated erythritol

Grated zest of ½ orange

1 teaspoon ground cinnamon

½ teaspoon Celtic sea salt

ALMOND CRUMBLE

½ cup almond flour

⅓ cup coconut flour

¼ cup sliced almonds

2 tablespoons brown sugar erythritol

4 tablespoons cold unsalted grass-fed butter, cubed

1 large egg, beaten

½ teaspoon almond extract

1. Preheat the oven to 375°F. Spray an 8 x 8-inch baking dish with cooking spray.

2. MAKE THE CRANBERRY-CHERRY FILLING: In a large bowl, toss together the cherries, cranberries, granulated erythritol, orange zest, cinnamon, and salt.

3. MAKE THE ALMOND CRUMBLE: In a medium bowl, combine the almond flour, coconut flour, sliced almonds, and brown sugar erythritol. Add the butter and pinch with your fingers until pea-sized crumbles form. Partway through pinching, add the egg and almond extract to evenly distribute.

4. Scrape the cherry filling into the prepared dish. Top with the crumble and bake until the topping is golden brown and the filling is bubbling, 20 to 25 minutes. Cool for 5 minutes before serving.

TIP: If prepping in advance, refrigerate the topping and the crumble in separate bowls until ready to bake.

PER SERVING ★ CALORIES: 172 ★ GRAMS OF PROTEIN: 4 ★ GRAMS OF FAT: 12 ★ GRAMS OF CARBOHYDRATE: 12 ★ PERCENT OF PROTEIN: 9% ★ PERCENT OF FAT: 63% ★ PERCENT OF CARBOHYDRATE: 28%

COCONUT CHIA BLUEBERRY PUDDING

PREP TIME: 5 MINUTES + OVERNIGHT REFRIGERATION ★ SERVINGS: 6

Chia seeds are rich in a super healthy fiber that helps with blood sugar, cholesterol regulation, digestive health, and more. In the past several years, they have proven deliciously worthy in puddings because of their ability to expand in liquid. Chia puddings fill you up and supply protein and healthy fats. I've been concocting chia puddings for years. The one you're about to dip your spoon into is my all-time favorite.

1½ cups blueberries

⅔ cup chia seeds

1 (14-ounce) can full-fat unsweetened coconut milk

1 cup heavy cream

½ teaspoon vanilla extract

½ teaspoon coconut extract

1 teaspoon grated lemon zest

¼ cup brown sugar erythritol

½ cup unsweetened coconut flakes, toasted, for garnish

1. In a food processor, pulse the blueberries until smooth. Transfer the puree to a large bowl and fold in the chia seeds, coconut milk, cream, vanilla, coconut extract, lemon zest, and erythritol to combine. Cover the bowl with plastic wrap and refrigerate overnight to firm up.

2. Serve sprinkled with the toasted coconut flakes.

PER SERVING ★ CALORIES: 319 ★ GRAMS OF PROTEIN: 5 ★ GRAMS OF FAT: 28 ★ GRAMS OF CARBOHYDRATE: 13 ★ PERCENT OF PROTEIN: 6% ★ PERCENT OF FAT: 78% ★ PERCENT OF CARBOHYDRATE: 16%

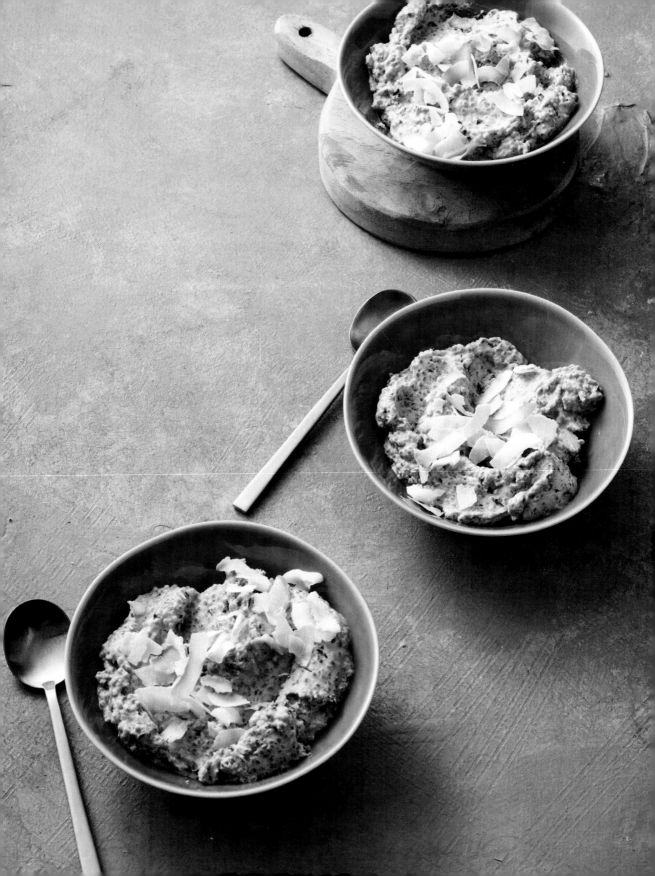

SHOPPING LISTS

The shopping lists that follow cover Tiers 2 and 3 of the plan and the recipes they contain, along with suggested amounts for each food item. How much you'll buy depends on whether you're cooking for just yourself or your family. You'll buy a lot less if you're cooking for one.

If you have leftovers, save them and freeze for another meal. Save time by cooking extra vegetables or protein or whatever you are having for your evening meal, so you can use the leftovers either for lunch or as a quicker meal the next evening. Soup can be made up to a week ahead and frozen.

Study the meal plans, and figure out which recipes you'll make, as well as any throw-together meals. Meal planning is important so that you purchase exactly what you need and don't overspend.

STAPLES (TO HAVE ON HAND)

Almond butter: 13-ounce jar

Almond flour: several 16-ounce bags

Apple cider vinegar: 32 fluid ounces

Baking powder

Broth (chicken or vegetable): 76 fluid ounces, or more

Butter, unsalted grass-fed: 1 pound

Cocoa powder, unsweetened

Coconut aminos: 16 fluid ounces

Coconut flour: 16-ounce bag

Coconut oil: 17 fluid ounces

Dijon mustard: 12 ounces

Ghee: 13-ounce jar

Grapeseed oil: 4 quarts

Hot sauce: 12 fluid ounces

Mayonnaise: 48-ounce jar

MCT oil: 17 fluid ounces

Olive oil, extra-virgin: 32 fluid ounces

Olive oil or avocado oil cooking spray

Peanut butter, creamy unsweetened natural: 36-ounce jar

Psyllium husk powder: 16-ounce bag

Red wine vinegar: 17 fluid ounces

Sesame oil: 17 fluid ounces

Tahini: 13-ounce jar

Xanthan gum

SPICES AND FLAVORINGS (TO HAVE ON HAND)

Adobo seasoning (such as Goya)

Almond extract

Black peppercorns, for grinding

Cayenne pepper

Celery seeds

Chili powder

Cinnamon

Coconut extract

Coriander, ground

Cumin, ground

Erythritol, brown sugar: 12-ounce package

Erythritol, confectioners': 12-ounce package

Erythritol, granulated: 12-ounce package

Garam masala

Garlic powder

Lemon-pepper

Nutmeg

Onion powder

Oregano, dried

Paprika, Hungarian sweet

Paprika, smoked

Paprika, sweet

Red pepper flakes

Rosemary, dried

Sea salt, Celtic

Stevia, granulated: 12-ounce package

Stevia, liquid: 2 ounces

Thyme, dried

Turmeric

Vanilla extract

White pepper, ground

TIER 2—WEEK 1

VEGETABLES

Bean sprouts: 6-ounce carton

Bell pepper, green: 1

Bibb lettuce: 2 heads

Broccoli: 1 cup florets

Butternut squash: 1

Cauliflower: 3 large heads

Celery: 1 bunch

Coleslaw mix: 1 bag

Cucumber, English: 1

Garlic: 2 bulbs

Ginger: 1 root

Leek: 1

Mustard greens: 8 cups
(1 pound)

Onion, red: 1 small

Onion, yellow: 2 small

Romaine lettuce: 2 heads

Scallions: 12

Shallot: 1

Tomato: 1 large

Watercress: 3 cups

Zucchini: 3 medium

FRESH HERBS

Basil: 1 package

Chives: 1 package

Cilantro: 1 package

Dill: 1 package

Mint: 1 package

Parsley: 1 bunch

Sage: 1 package

Thyme: 1 package

FRUITS

Avocado: 2

Lemons: 8 to 10

Limes: 2

PROTEINS

Bacon: 1 pound

Beef, ground: 2 pounds +
12 ounces
(preferably grass-fed)

Chicken breasts, boneless,
skinless: 2 (8-ounce) breasts

Chicken thighs, boneless,
skinless: 1 pound

Eggs, large: 2 dozen

Fish (such as halibut):
4 (6-ounce) fillets

Flank steak: 1½ pounds
(preferably grass-fed)

Salmon, wild: 1 pound skinless
fillets

Steaks, sirloin: 4 (6-ounce) cuts
(preferably grass-fed)

Tuna: 4 (5-ounce) cans
water-packed light

CHEESE AND OTHER DAIRY

Blue cheese crumbles:
8-ounce tub

Cheddar cheese, sharp,
shredded: 8-ounce package

Cream, heavy: 1 pint

Feta cheese, crumbled:
8-ounce tub

Greek yogurt, whole-milk, plain:
6-ounce container

Mozzarella cheese, whole-milk:
4 ounces

Parmesan cheese, shredded:
8-ounce package

Parmigiano-Reggiano cheese,
grated: 8-ounce tub

NUTS AND SEEDS

Almonds: 16-ounce package

Mixed nuts: 34-ounce jar

Sesame seeds: 1-ounce
container

OTHER

Kalamata olives: 9.5-ounce jar

Marinara sauce, no-sugar-
added: 25-ounce jar

Pork rinds: 8.5-ounce bag

Tomatoes, crushed:
28-ounce can

Whisps: 9.5-ounce bag

TIER 2—WEEK 2

VEGETABLES

Baby bok choy: 4 heads

Bell pepper, green: 1

Bibb lettuce: 1 or 2 heads

Brussels sprouts: 1 pound

Cabbage, red: 1 small head

Cauliflower: 3 large heads

Cremini mushrooms: 1 cup

Garlic: 1 bulb

Onion, yellow: 3 small

Romaine lettuce: 2 heads

Scallions: 6

Shallot: 1

Spinach, baby: 4 cups

Zucchini noodles, store-bought: 1 pound

FRESH HERBS

Chives: 1 package

Cilantro: 1 package

Parsley: 1 bunch

Thyme: 1 package

FRUITS

Avocado: 1

Blueberries: 6-ounce carton (freeze leftover berries)

Lemons: 10 to 12

Limes: 6

Raspberries: 6-ounce carton (freeze leftover berries)

Strawberries, frozen, unsweetened: 16-ounce bag

PROTEINS

Bacon: 1 pound

Beef, ground: 2 pounds + 12 ounces (preferably grass-fed)

Chicken tenders: 1 pound

Chicken thighs, boneless, skinless: ½ pound

Cod: 1½ pounds skinless fillets

Eggs, large: 2 dozen

Pepperoni slices: ¼ cup

Pork chop, sirloin, 1 to 4 (6-ounce) cuts

Pork, ground: 1 pound

Steaks, sirloin: 1 to 4 (6-ounce) cuts (preferably grass-fed)

Sweet Italian sausage links: 2

Veal, ground: ½ pound

CHEESE AND OTHER DAIRY

Buttermilk, full-fat: 1 quart

Cheddar cheese, sharp, shredded: 8-ounce package

Coconut milk, full-fat unsweetened: 1 can

Cream cheese, full-fat: 4 ounces

Cream, heavy: 1 pint

Milk, whole: 1 pint

Mozzarella cheese, low-moisture whole-milk, shredded: 3 (8-ounce) packages

Parmesan cheese, shredded: 8-ounce package

Parmigiano-Reggiano cheese, grated: 8-ounce tub

NUTS AND SEEDS

Chia seeds: 8-ounce bag

Pumpkin seeds (pepitas): ⅓ cup

OTHER

Chili-garlic sauce: 18-ounce jar

Marinara sauce, no-sugar-added: 25-ounce jar

Pork rinds: 8.5-ounce bag

Sun-dried tomatoes: 8.5-ounce jar

Tomatoes, crushed: 28-ounce can

Tomato paste: 6-ounce can

Tomato puree: 15-ounce can

Vanilla protein powder (such as Isopure): 1 (3-pound) carton

Whisps: 9.5-ounce bag

TIER 2—WEEK 3

VEGETABLES

Artichokes: 16-ounce can packed in water

Arugula, baby: 5-ounce box

Bean sprouts: 6-ounce carton

Bell pepper, red: 1

Bell pepper, yellow: 1

Bibb lettuce: 2 heads

Broccoli: 2 cups florets

Cabbage, green: 1 small head

Cabbage, red: 1 small head

Cauliflower: 2 large heads

Celery: 1 bunch

Cremini mushrooms: 8 ounces

Cucumber, English: 3

Garlic: 1 bulb

Ginger: 1 root

Jalapeños: 6

Kale, baby: 3 cups

Onion, red: 2 small

Onion, yellow: 2 small

Romaine lettuce: 1 head

Scallions: 6

Shallots: 3

Shiitake mushrooms: 8 ounces

Spinach, baby: 3 cups

Spinach, frozen: 14 ounces

Tomato: 1 large

Watercress: 3 cups

Zucchini: 3 medium

FRESH HERBS

Basil: 1 package

Chives: 1 package

Cilantro: 1 package

Dill: 1 package

Mint: 1 package

Parsley: 1 bunch

FRUITS

Avocado: 1

Lemons: 12

Limes: 12

PROTEINS

Bacon: 1 pound

Beef, ground: 2½ pounds (preferably grass-fed)

Chicken thighs, boneless, skinless: 4 (6-ounce) thighs + ¾ pound

Eggs, large: ½ dozen

Pork, ground: ¾ pound

Salmon, wild: 2 pounds skinless fillets

Shrimp: 1 pound

Skirt steak: 1 pound (preferably grass-fed)

Tuna: 4 (5-ounce) cans water-packed light

Veal, ground: ½ pound

CHEESE AND OTHER DAIRY

Cheddar cheese, sharp, shredded: 2 (8-ounce) packages

Coconut milk, full-fat unsweetened: 1 can

Cream cheese, full-fat: 16 ounces

Cream, heavy: 2 pints

Feta cheese, crumbled: 8-ounce tub

Greek yogurt, whole-milk, plain: 6-ounce container

Milk, whole: 1 pint

Mozzarella cheese, whole-milk: 8 ounces

Parmesan cheese, shredded: 8-ounce package

Parmigiano-Reggiano cheese, grated: 8-ounce tub

NUTS AND SEEDS

Peanuts, roasted, salted: 12-ounce jar

Pistachios, shelled: ¼ cup

Pomegranate seeds: ¼ cup

Pumpkin seeds (pepitas): ⅓ cup

OTHER

Anchovy paste: 1.6-ounce container

Fish sauce: 24 fluid ounces

Shirataki noodles: 2 (7-ounce) bags

Sriracha: 17-ounce container

Tomatoes, crushed: 28-ounce can

Tomato paste: 6-ounce can

Tomato puree: 15-ounce can

Whisps: 9.5-ounce bag

TIER 3—WEEK 1

VEGETABLES

Bean sprouts: 6-ounce carton

Bell pepper, green: 1

Bibb lettuce: 1 head

Broccoli: 3 cups florets

Cauliflower: 1 head

Garlic: 1 clove

Ginger: 1 root

Kale, baby: ½ cup

Onion, yellow: 1 small

Romaine lettuce: 2 heads

Scallions: 2

Shallot: 1

Spinach, baby: 5 cups

Spinach, frozen: 14 ounces

Tomato: 1 large

Watercress: 3 cups

FRESH HERBS

Basil: 1 package

Chives: 1 package

Cilantro: 1 package

Dill: 1 package

Parsley: 1 bunch

FRUITS

Avocado: 2

Cantaloupe chunks, frozen:
¼ cup

Cherries, pitted, frozen,
unsweetened: ¼ cup

Cranberries, frozen,
unsweetened: 1½ cups

Lemons: 9

Limes: 4

Mixed berries, unsweetened,
frozen: ½ cup

Orange (for zesting): 1

Strawberries: 6-ounce carton
(freeze leftover berries)

PROTEINS

Bacon: 1 pound

Beef, ground: 3½ pounds
(preferably grass-fed)

Chicken breasts, boneless,
skinless: 4 (8-ounce) breasts

Chicken tenders: ½ pound

Chicken thighs, boneless,
skinless: 1 pound

Egg, large: 1

Fish (halibut): 4 (6-ounce)
skinless fillets

Flank steak: 1½ pounds
(preferably grass-fed)

Shrimp, medium-large:
1½ pounds

Steaks, sirloin: 1 to 4 (6-ounce)
cuts (preferably grass-fed)

Tuna: 4 (5-ounce) cans
water-packed light

CHEESE AND OTHER DAIRY

Blue cheese crumbles:
8-ounce tub

Buttermilk, full-fat: 1 quart

Cheddar cheese, sharp,
shredded: 2 (8-ounce)
packages

Coconut milk, full-fat
unsweetened: 1 can

Cream cheese, full-fat:
4 ounces

Cream, heavy: 1 to 2 pints

Greek yogurt, whole-milk, plain:
6-ounce container

Milk, whole: 1 pint

Mozzarella cheese, low-
moisture whole-milk, shredded:
16 ounces

Mozzarella cheese, whole-milk:
4 ounces

Parmesan cheese, shredded:
8-ounce package

Parmigiano-Reggiano cheese,
grated: 8-ounce tub

Ricotta cheese, whole-milk:
1¼ cups

Sour cream: 8 ounces

OTHER

Marinara sauce, no-sugar-
added: 25-ounce jar

Pork rinds: 8.5-ounce bag

Stevia-sweetened dark
chocolate baking chips
(such as Lily's): 9-ounce bag

Tomato puree: 15-ounce can

Whisps: 9.5-ounce bag

TIER 3—WEEK 2

VEGETABLES

Baby bok choy: 6 heads

Bean sprouts: 6-ounce carton

Bell pepper, green: 1

Bell pepper, red: 1

Bibb lettuce: 1 head

Broccoli: 3 cups florets

Brussels sprouts: 1 pound

Cabbage, red: 1 small head

Carrot: 1

Cauliflower: 4 heads

Celery: 1 bunch

Garlic: 1 bulb

Ginger: 1 root

Kale, baby: ½ cup

Onion, yellow: 2 small

Romaine lettuce: 3 heads

Scallions: 8

Shallot: 1

Spinach, baby: 2 cups

FRESH HERBS

Chives: 1 package

Cilantro: 1 package

Parsley: 1 bunch

Thyme: 1 package

FRUITS

Avocado: 4

Blueberries: 6-ounce carton (freeze leftover berries)

Lemons: 7 to 10

Limes: 9

Raspberries, frozen: 1 small carton (freeze leftover berries)

PROTEINS

Bacon: 1 pound

Beef, ground: 1½ pounds + 12 ounces (preferably grass-fed)

Chicken tenders: 1 pound

Chicken thighs, boneless, skinless: ½ pound

Chorizo: 6 ounces

Cod: 1½ pounds skinless fillets

Eggs, large: 2½ dozen

Pepperoni slices: ¼ cup

Pork chop, sirloin: 1 to 4 (6-ounce) cuts

Pork, ground: ½ pound

Steaks, sirloin: 2 to 8 (6-ounce) cuts (preferably grass-fed)

Sweet Italian sausage links: 2

CHEESE AND OTHER DAIRY

Blue cheese crumbles: 8-ounce tub

Buttermilk, full-fat: 1 quart

Cheddar cheese, sharp, shredded: 8-ounce package

Coconut milk, full-fat unsweetened: 2 (14-ounce) cans

Cream cheese, full-fat: 4 ounces

Cream, heavy: 1 quart

Greek yogurt, whole-milk, plain: 6-ounce container

Milk, whole: 1 pint

Mozzarella cheese, whole-milk, grated: 16 ounces

Parmesan cheese, shredded: 1½ cups

Parmigiano-Reggiano cheese, grated: 8-ounce tub

Ricotta cheese, whole-milk: 1 cup

Sour cream: 8 ounces

NUTS AND SEEDS

Coconut flakes, unsweetened: 16-ounce package

Macadamia nuts: 6.25-ounce jar

Pecan halves: 24-ounce bag

Pumpkin seeds (pepitas): 2-ounce package

Sunflower seeds: 2-ounce package

OTHER

Marinara sauce, no-sugar-added: 25-ounce jar

Pork rinds: 8.5-ounce bag

Stevia-sweetened dark chocolate baking chips (such as Lily's): 9-ounce bag

Tomato puree: 15-ounce can

TIER 3—WEEK 3

VEGETABLES

Arugula, baby: 5-ounce box

Bean sprouts: 6-ounce carton

Bell pepper, red: 1

Bell pepper, yellow: 1

Bibb lettuce: 1 head

Broccoli: 2 cups florets

Cabbage, green: 1 small head

Cabbage, red: 1 small head

Cauliflower: 2 heads

Cucumber, English: 2

Eggplant: 1 (1 pound 3 ounces)

Garlic: 1 bulb

Ginger: 1 root

Jalapeños: 6

Kale, baby: 4 cups

Onion, red: 1 small

Onion, yellow: 5 small

Scallions: 6

Shallot: 1

Shiitake mushrooms: 8 ounces

Spinach, baby: 3 cups

Spinach, frozen: 2 (10-ounce) packages

Zucchini: 2 large or 3 small

FRESH HERBS

Basil: 1 package

Chives: 1 package

Cilantro: 1 package

Dill: 1 package

Mint: 1 package

Parsley: 1 bunch

FRUITS

Avocado: 3

Blueberries: 6-ounce carton (freeze leftover berries)

Lemons: 2

Limes: 8

Mixed berries, unsweetened, frozen: ½ cup

PROTEINS

Bacon: 1 pound

Beef chuck: 4 ounces + 2 pounds (preferably grass-fed)

Beef, ground: 2 pounds (preferably grass-fed)

Breakfast sausage: ½ pound

Chicken thighs, boneless, skinless: ¾ pound + 4 (6-ounce) thighs

Eggs, large: 2 dozen

Pepperoni slices: ¼ cup

Pork, ground: ½ pound

Salmon, wild: 2 pounds skinless fillets

Shrimp: 1 pound

Skirt steak: 1 pound (preferably grass-fed)

Steaks, sirloin: 4 (6-ounce) cuts (preferably grass-fed)

Sweet Italian sausage links: 2

CHEESE AND OTHER DAIRY

Cheddar cheese, sharp, shredded: 2 (8-ounce) packages

Coconut cream, unsweetened: 5.4-ounce can

Coconut milk, full-fat, unsweetened: 2 (14-ounce) cans

Cream cheese, full-fat: 8 ounces

Cream, heavy: 1 quart

Feta cheese, crumbled: 8-ounce tub

Greek yogurt, whole-milk, plain: 2 (6-ounce) containers

Milk, whole: 1 pint

Mozzarella cheese, low-moisture whole-milk, shredded: 16 ounces

Parmigiano-Reggiano cheese, grated: 8-ounce tub

Ricotta cheese, whole-milk: 8 ounces

NUTS AND SEEDS

Almonds: 1 cup

Coconut flakes, unsweetened: 16-ounce package

Macadamia nuts: 6.25-ounce jar

Peanuts, roasted, salted: ⅓ cup

Pistachios, shelled: ¼ cup

Pomegranate seeds: ¼ cup

Poppy seeds: 2.6-ounce jar

Pumpkin seeds (pepitas): 1½ cups

Sunflower seeds: ½ cup

OTHER

Marinara sauce, no-sugar-added: 25-ounce jar

Pork rinds: 8.5-ounce bag

Shirataki noodles: 2 (7-ounce) bags

Stevia-sweetened dark chocolate baking chips (such as Lily's): 9-ounce bag

Tomatoes, canned, crushed: 1 cup

Tomatoes, chopped: 28-ounce can

Tomato paste: 6-ounce can

Tomato puree: 15-ounce can

Whisps: 9.5-ounce bag

EATING OUT, KETO COMFORT—STYLE

As much as I love to cook, I also enjoy eating out. I'm a member of the huge club of Americans who are eating out more frequently than ever. In the United States alone, the average family spends nearly $3,000 on meals away from home each year, according to the National Restaurant Association.

If you're shifting over to keto dieting, you may be wondering what you can eat at restaurants or if you can dine out at all. Maybe you think that if you do eat out, you have to stick with a boring, no-dressing salad or chicken breast and steamed veggies. Not true.

With the Keto Comfort Food Diet, it's easy to dine anywhere—restaurants, airports, sporting events, on vacations—and stay in ketosis. All you have to do is follow two simple rules:

RULE #1: ENJOY PROTEINS, FAT-RICH FOODS, AND NONSTARCHY VEGETABLES

☐ Meats like steak, chicken, pork, lamb, bacon, and sausage (no breading)

☐ Seafood, all varieties of fish and shellfish (no breading)

☐ Nonstarchy vegetables, especially salad veggies and cruciferous vegetables

☐ Lettuce wraps in place of breads and buns

☐ Eggs, prepared any way you desire

☐ Small cheese plates

☐ Condiments, including olive oil, butter, vinegar, and salad dressings like blue cheese

☐ Nuts and seeds as toppings

RULE #2: AVOID STARCHY CARBS AND SUGARY SWEETS

☐ Noodles and pastas, even whole-grain and soba varieties

☐ Grains like rice, quinoa, oats, grits, cereals, barley, millet, and couscous

☐ Tortillas and chips (dipping celery sticks in guacamole tastes divine)

☐ French fries, sweet potato fries, or any breaded, fried veggie

☐ Breads

☐ Sweet sauces and condiments such as sweet and sour sauce and ketchup

☐ Starchy vegetables like potatoes, sweet potatoes, carrots, parsnips, most winter squashes, beans, and legumes

☐ Desserts with the exception of fresh berries with cream

If you want more specifics, here's a roster of all sorts of restaurants, each with a list of sample meals you can order—plus what to avoid. Plan ahead and identify keto-friendly food choices so you don't give in to impulse ordering.

AMERICAN-STYLE CHAIN RESTAURANTS
(SUCH AS APPLEBEE'S, CHILI'S, RUBY TUESDAY, AND TGI FRIDAYS)

Chain restaurants offer lots of keto choices.

1. Grilled sirloin with portobello mushrooms or roasted tomatoes, avocado, and mixed greens with oil and vinegar dressing

2. Grilled chicken salad with oil and vinegar dressing

3. Seafood salad with oil and vinegar dressing

4. Grilled or blackened salmon with broccoli, or any fresh fish dinner with seasonal vegetables and a garden salad with oil and vinegar dressing

5. Grilled or blackened chicken with steamed vegetables and salad with oil and vinegar dressing

6. Grilled turkey burger and steamed broccoli

7. "Unwich" (a lettuce-wrapped burger or sandwich)

WHAT TO AVOID: Fried entrées, burgers on buns, sandwiches, and anything laden with sauces

ASIAN RESTAURANTS

When I was a kid growing up in the Jamaica neighborhood of Queens, my family often went to an Asian take-out place close to our house. Asian food is near and dear to my heart. I love it even more these days because it is so easy to customize to a weight-loss diet. Here are some suggestions for what to order while you're following the Keto Comfort Food Diet.

1. Carb-free lettuce wraps, made with chicken, red onions, nuts, and other vegetables

2. Soup (healthy choices include broth-based soups such as egg drop, miso, or hot and sour soup) and seaweed salad

3. Steamed dishes, without noodles or rice or sauces (which are rich in cornstarch)

4. Sashimi and a seaweed salad, cucumber salad, or simple house salad with oil and vinegar dressing on the side

5. Chicken or beef (not fried or breaded) with steamed vegetables (no sugary or starchy sauces)

6. Vegetable-based entrées if steamed or stir-fried using a minimal amount of oil

7. Moo shu (vegetables, chicken, and shrimp) without pancakes

8. Crispy duck without sweet and sour sauce

9. Stir-fries made with meat, poultry, seafood, and nonstarchy vegetables—without the rice and sauce

WHAT TO AVOID: Spareribs, General Tso's chicken, egg rolls, fried wontons, fried rice, orange chicken, sesame chicken, sweet and sour entrées, fried entrées, and anything coated with a sticky, heavy sweet sauce

BARBECUE RESTAURANTS

Here comes a meat-head's dream: barbecue. Because barbecue emphasizes fat and protein, you can enjoy this stuff without slipping out of ketosis.

When you think of barbecue joints, you probably think juicy, meaty "ribs." It doesn't get much better than that, don't you agree? But if you eat too many, you'll barely be able to see or touch your own. Even so, don't be afraid to venture into a barbecue restaurant. With so many grilled proteins on the menu, there's a lot you can eat without packing on the pounds.

1. Brisket served with a simple salt-and-pepper rub and a side of green beans—most important: no sugary sauce!

2. Roasted chicken and a side of green beans or broccoli

3. Char-grilled chicken breast and a side of green beans or vinegar-based (not creamy) coleslaw

4. Grilled or blackened shrimp and a simple house salad with oil and vinegar dressing

5. Blackened catfish and a simple house salad with oil and vinegar dressing

6. Smoked barbecue turkey and vinegar-based (not creamy) coleslaw, sliced onion, and dill pickle

7. Pulled pork and vinegar-based (not creamy) coleslaw, sliced onion, and dill pickle

8. Grilled sausage with smoked green beans or collard greens

9. Southwestern grilled pork tenderloin and nonstarchy veggies

10. Grilled butterflied leg of lamb and a side salad with oil and vinegar dressing

11. Blackened salmon and green beans or a simple house salad with oil and vinegar dressing on the side

WHAT TO AVOID: Spareribs, fried entrées, sandwiches, and anything laden with barbecue sauce

BREAKFAST RESTAURANTS

I love eating breakfast out. Have someone serve me piping-hot espresso, scrambled eggs, and bacon (hold the buttery toast), and I'm in food heaven. With keto dieting, you can enjoy lots of cream in your coffee, too. Here are your best keto bets for breakfast.

1. Vegetable omelet with spinach, tomatoes, and mushrooms

2. Scrambled eggs with vegetables (such as spinach, tomatoes, and mushrooms)

3. Scrambled eggs with bacon, sausage, or ham

4. Bacon and fresh berries

5. Greek yogurt, with a sprinkling of nuts, and fresh berries

6. Scrambled eggs and a sliced tomato

7. Smoked salmon (lox), cream cheese, and fresh berries

8. Sausage and sliced tomatoes or fresh berries

9. Cheese omelet

10. Steak and eggs

WHAT TO AVOID: Cereals, hash browns, pancakes, waffles, bagels, doughnuts, and crepes

DELI RESTAURANTS

I love delis. Being a New Yorker, I grew up with them, and the food never goes out of style. And there's plenty of it—including numerous choices that fit right into the keto lifestyle.

1. Additive-free turkey or chicken deli meat and vinegar-based (not creamy) coleslaw

2. Low-fat beef deli meat or hot corned beef and vinegar-based (not creamy) coleslaw

3. Broth-based soups such as chicken or vegetable

4. All-vegetable salad: choose a leafy green base and pile your favorite fresh nonstarchy veggies as high as you like

5. Grilled chicken salad with oil and vinegar dressing on the side

6. Plate of steamed nonstarchy veggies

7. Smoked salmon (lox) salad with oil and vinegar dressing

8. Entrée salad, such as a chef's salad, with oil and vinegar dressing on the side

WHAT TO AVOID: Sandwiches made with breads and fried entrées

FAST FOOD

I'll probably go to chef hell for even mentioning fast-food restaurants, but there are some good choices that let you eat fast food and still stay true to a keto diet.

1. Southwestern or taco salad (without the shell)

2. Chicken Caesar garden salad

3. Grilled or blackened chicken breast, green beans, and vinegar-based (not creamy) coleslaw (at a fried chicken establishment)

4. Grilled chicken and a side salad with oil and vinegar dressing

5. Rotisserie chicken and steamed vegetables

6. Any broiled hamburger (toss out the bun) and a side salad with oil and vinegar dressing

7. Salad bar entrée salad: choose nonstarchy vegetables and lean protein

8. Roast beef (skip the bun or bread) and a side salad with oil and vinegar dressing

9. Charbroiled turkey burger (skip the bun) and a side salad with oil and vinegar dressing

10. Baked fish and steamed vegetables

WHAT TO AVOID: Everything except what I've listed!

FRENCH RESTAURANTS

If I was on death row and had to order my last meal, it would be a French dish, swimming in cheese sauce. But before my mouth starts watering too much, let me say that you shouldn't be intimidated by French food. A lot of French food is really not that rich in carbs and can be worked into the Keto Comfort Food Diet any day of the week.

1. Bouillabaisse (a broth-based fish stew)

2. Salmon tartare and a salad with a light vinegar-based dressing

3. Any roasted meat or poultry and a vegetable salad with oil and vinegar dressing

4. Any braised meat or poultry and a vegetable salad with oil and vinegar dressing

5. Grilled fish and a vegetable salad with oil and vinegar dressing

6. Steak au poivre and a vegetable salad with oil and vinegar dressing

7. Salade niçoise (skip the potatoes and ask for extra green beans instead)

8. Grilled frog legs and a vegetable salad with oil and vinegar dressing

9. Beef bourguignon with sautéed vegetables

WHAT TO AVOID: Breaded, fried, and sauced entrées

GREEK RESTAURANTS

I adore Greek food, and the world can't have enough Greek restaurants, in my opinion. You can rarely go wrong at a Greek restaurant with its cuisine rich in vegetables and lean protein.

1. Vegetable kebabs

2. Souvlaki (kebabs made of chicken, lamb, or pork)

3. Charbroiled portobello mushrooms, zucchini, peppers, onions, and tomatoes, served with a small Greek salad with oil and vinegar dressing

4. Dinner-sized Greek salad

5. Goat cheese, olives, and Greek salad with tomatoes

6. Grilled lamb chops and a small Greek salad

7. Gyros (without the bread) and a small Greek salad

8. Kakavia (a traditional Greek fisherman's soup typically made with the catch of the day or whatever is seasonal, like snapper, mullet, or whitefish)

9. Any seafood meal that is grilled, pan-seared, or broiled (not fried) and offers a side of fresh vegetables or salad

10. For dessert, goat's milk yogurt with some lemon juice and cinnamon (consider adding your own stevia)

WHAT TO AVOID: Moussaka, stuffed grape leaves (unless they're made without rice), spinach pie, and baklava

INDIAN RESTAURANTS

When I'm not working in my own kitchen and have a rare evening off, I like to drop by an Indian restaurant. Like most ethnic foods, Indian cuisine includes lots of animal protein and vegetables and is prepared with ghee (clarified butter), which is allowed on my plan. There are plenty of healthy selections you can make and still protect your precious ketosis.

1. Tandoori chicken, lamb, or shrimp

2. Curried fish as long as it isn't breaded and fried

3. Roasted eggplant with onions and spices

4. Curried vegetables

5. Chicken tikka (very similar to tandoori but boneless)

6. Chicken korma (but double-check ingredients as preparations can differ)

7. Indian kebabs

8. Spinach soup with a dab of ghee

9. Shahi paneer (a homemade cheese in a curried tomato sauce)

10. Chicken shorba (chicken soup made with garlic, ginger, cinnamon, cumin, and other spices)

WHAT TO AVOID: Fried or fat-laden bread (pappadum, chapati, naan, kulcha, or roti), heavily fried entrées, and starchy dishes like rice

ITALIAN RESTAURANTS

Your friends want to meet at an Italian restaurant and the dialogue in your head starts: "How am I going to manage eating well with all that pasta?" Here's how, with these keto-friendly and delicious choices. Always check to see if you can substitute spaghetti squash for pasta.

1. Tuscan grilled steak and a side salad with oil and vinegar dressing

2. Chicken cacciatore (without the pasta)

3. Minestrone without noodles and a side salad with oil and vinegar dressing

4. Caesar salad with grilled chicken or shrimp and dressing

5. Cold vegetable salads, drizzled with a little olive oil, or antipasto salads

6. Grilled chicken and a side salad with oil and vinegar dressing, or a tomato-cucumber salad

7. Grilled fish and a side salad with oil and vinegar dressing, or a tomato-mozzarella (caprese) salad

8. Grilled veal and a side salad with oil and vinegar dressing, or a tomato-cucumber salad

9. Chicken or veal marsala and a side salad with oil and vinegar dressing, or a tomato-mozzarella (caprese) salad

10. Lightly sautéed squid (no breading) with a side of Italian vegetables such as grilled zucchini or eggplant

WHAT TO AVOID: Entrées made with pastas such as fettuccine Alfredo, ravioli, lasagna, and spaghetti with meatballs; chicken or eggplant or veal parmigiana (usually breaded); garlic bread; and gnocchi

MEXICAN RESTAURANTS

The ever-present and bottomless tortilla chips, cheese, and high-calorie margaritas give Mexican restaurants an undeserved negative reputation. But the fact is, Mexican food *can* be enjoyed while you're on the Keto Comfort Food Diet.

1. Fish steamed and covered with fresh tomatillo sauce

2. Grilled fish and a side salad with oil and vinegar dressing

3. Mexican-seasoned grilled chicken with a side of vinegar-based (not creamy) coleslaw and pico de gallo

4. Ceviche (shrimp, scallops, and fish marinated in lime juice)

5. Chicken, beef, or shrimp fajitas—hold the tortillas

6. Gazpacho (spicy vegetable soup served cool)

7. Taco salad—skip the deep-fried, bowl-shaped tortilla

8. Carnitas (marinated grilled beef strips) and a side salad with oil and vinegar dressing or a vinegar-based (not creamy) coleslaw

WHAT TO AVOID: Entrées labeled *grande, supreme,* or *combo;* fried foods like tortilla chips; chimichangas; and burritos

STEAKHOUSES

Steakhouses are a keto dieter's delight because of the protein choices. Veer toward filet mignon, sirloin, chicken, or fish, paired up with veggies. But watch your protein portion sizes. You don't have to eat the whole animal.

1. Filet mignon or petite sirloin, nonstarchy vegetable medley, and a tossed side salad with oil and vinegar or blue cheese dressing

2. Grilled chicken breast, nonstarchy vegetable medley, and a tossed side salad with oil and vinegar or blue cheese dressing

3. Grilled salmon or tilapia, nonstarchy vegetable medley, and a tossed side salad with oil and vinegar or blue cheese dressing

4. Lobster tails or snow crab legs, nonstarchy vegetable medley, and a tossed side salad with oil and vinegar or blue cheese dressing

5. Grilled shrimp, nonstarchy vegetable medley, and a tossed side salad with oil and vinegar or blue cheese dressing

6. Large ahi tuna appetizer and a tossed side salad with oil and vinegar dressing

7. Any entrée salad or salad bar salad, but skip the croutons

8. Grilled kebabs made with beef, chicken, or shrimp and nonstarchy vegetables such as bell peppers, tomatoes, and mushrooms

9. Plate of various types of steamed nonstarchy veggies

10. Shrimp cocktail (with hot sauce but no cocktail sauce) and a tossed side salad with oil and vinegar dressing

WHAT TO AVOID: Huge portions of meat such as rib eye or prime rib; breaded and fried foods; any food smothered in sauce; starchy sides such as mashed potatoes and steak fries

No matter which cuisine you choose, it's good to know what's on the menu before you go. Check online to see what's keto-friendly—grilled protein entrées, salads, vegetable sides, and so on. I've found that it's pretty easy to stick to the Keto Comfort Food Diet at most establishments. Once you practice these keto comfort food strategies a few times, you'll create positive habits that will keep you in ketosis when eating out.

REFERENCES

Boschmann, M., et al. 2003. Water-induced thermogenesis. *The Journal of Clinical Endocrinology and Metabolism* 88:6015–6019.

Brietzke, E., et al. 2018. Ketogenic diet as a metabolic therapy for mood disorders: Evidence and developments. *Neuroscience & Biobehavioral Reviews* 94:11–16.

Bueno, N. B., et al. 2013. Very-low-carbohydrate ketogenic diet v. low-fat diet for long-term weight loss: A meta-analysis of randomised controlled trials. *British Journal of Nutrition* 110:1178–1187.

Choi, Y., et al. 2013. Indole-3-carbinol directly targets SIRT1 to inhibit adipocyte differentiation. *International Journal of Obesity* 37: 881–884.

Dehghan, M., et al. 2017. Associations of fats and carbohydrate intake with cardiovascular disease and mortality in 18 countries from five continents (PURE): A prospective cohort study. *Lancet* 390:2050–2062.

Dennis, E. A., et al. 2010. Water consumption increases weight loss during a hypocaloric diet intervention in middle-aged and older adults. *Obesity* 18:300–307.

Gearhardt, A. N., et al. 2011. Neural correlates of food addiction. *Archives of General Psychiatry* 68:808–816.

Gibson, A. A., et al. 2016. Accuracy of hands v. household measures as portion size estimation aids. *Journal of Nutritional Science* 5:e29.

Goday, A., et al. 2016. Short-term safety, tolerability and efficacy of a very low-calorie-ketogenic diet interventional weight loss program versus hypocaloric diet in patients with type 2 diabetes mellitus. *Nutrition & Diabetes* 6:e230.

Gomez-Arbelaez, D., et al. 2018. Resting metabolic rate of obese patients under very low calorie ketogenic diet. *Nutrition & Metabolism* 15:18.

Hussain, T. A., et al. 2012. Effect of low-calorie versus low-carbohydrate ketogenic diet in type 2 diabetes. *Nutrition* 28:1016–1021.

Hyland, C., et al. 2019. Organic diet intervention significantly reduces urinary pesticide levels in U.S. children and adults. *Science Direct* 171:568–575.

Kearns, C. E., et al. 2016. Sugar industry and coronary heart disease research: A historical analysis of internal industry documents. *JAMA Internal Medicine* 176:1680–1685.

Köhnke, R., et al. 2009. Thylakoids promote release of the satiety hormone cholecystokinin while reducing insulin in healthy humans. *Scandinavian Journal of Gastroenterology* 44:712–719.

Moreno, B., et al. 2014. Comparison of a very-low-calorie-ketogenic diet with a standard low-calorie diet in the treatment of obesity. *Endocrine* 47: 793–805.

Myett-Côté, E., et al. 2018. Prior ingestion of exogenous ketone monoester attenuates the glycaemic response to an oral glucose tolerance test in healthy young individuals. *Journal of Physiology* 596:1385–1395.

Stubbs, B.J., et al. 2018. A ketone ester drink lowers human ghrelin and appetite. *Obesity* 26:269–273.

Vargas, S., et al. 2018. Efficacy of ketogenic diet on body composition during resistance training in trained men: A randomized controlled trial. *Journal of the International Society of Sports Nutrition* 15:31.

Vergati, M., et al. 2017. Ketogenic diet and other dietary intervention strategies in the treatment of cancer. *Current Medicinal Chemistry* 24: 1170–1185.

Walczyk, T., and J. Y. Wick. 2017. The ketogenic diet: Making a comeback. *The Consultant Pharmacist* 32:388–398.

Westman, E. C., et al. 2008. The effect of a low-carbohydrate, ketogenic diet versus a low-glycemic index diet on glycemic control in type 2 diabetes mellitus. *Nutrition & Metabolism* 5:36.

Yancy, W. S., Jr., et al. 2005. A low-carbohydrate, ketogenic diet to treat type 2 diabetes. *Nutrition & Metabolism* 2:34.

Yancy, W. S., Jr., et al. 2010. A randomized trial of a low-carbohydrate diet vs orlistat plus a low-fat diet for weight loss. *Archives of Internal Medicine* 170:136–145.

Zilberter, T., and E. Y. Zilberter. 2014. Breakfast: To skip or not to skip? *Frontiers in Public Health* 2:59.

ACKNOWLEDGMENTS

In a busy restaurant kitchen, the executive chef has a team of other chefs helping, including a sous-chef (the second in command) and line cooks, who are assigned a certain place in the food production process such as the grill, oven, or vegetable prep line, and many other assistants. It takes an entire group of talented people to make great cuisine happen—and this teamwork is similar to what happens in producing a book. So I'd like to thank my "chefs" on my book team for making this book happen: Diana, Michele, Celeste, Sarah, Anna, Maggie, Laura, Toby, and others behind the scenes who helped me create a book of which I'm proud and one that will help so many people get happier and healthier.